WIT

ON MY MIND

WITH YOU
ON MY MIND

A Personal Experience
of Caring for Someone with
Lewy Body Dementia

Brian Hallett

DISCLAIMER

Every care has been taken in the production of this book, but no legal responsibility is accepted, warranted or implied by the author and publisher in respect of any errors, omissions or misstatements. You should always seek professional advice from a suitably qualified person.

© Brian Hallett, 2018

Published by BH Books

A CIP catalogue record for this book is available from the British Library.

ISBN 978-0-9501640-0-7

Book layout and cover design by Clare Brayshaw

Prepared and printed by:

York Publishing Services Ltd
64 Hallfield Road
Layerthorpe
York YO31 7ZQ

Tel: 01904 431213

Website: www.yps-publishing.co.uk

PREFACE

In the autumn of 2013, my wife's occasional lapses of memory became sufficiently significant for me to make a reference to them in my diary.

Her sometimes dotty approach to life had always been an essential part of her charm, but it was early in the following year that it occurred to me that these lapses could be the onset of dementia. As her difficulties worsened, the diary entries became more frequent, and I was prompted to search for books on the subject – just in case.

Nothing came to light that seemed to match exactly what I was seeing, and this still seems to be the case. It occurs to me that my jottings might be the basis for a book that could help others in the same position and facing similar problems.

I am not a doctor; my only qualification is that I helped Jeanne along every inch of the twisting, tortuous path that changed her life, and mine, for ever. This is a layman's view of a life-changing illness of which little is known by the general public and about which it was hard to find useful information.

If someone you love has started to develop signs of dementia, this book may help you. If, as their main carer, you feel out of your depth, if you find yourself searching for answers, for advice, for reassurance and none is forthcoming – you and I have a lot in common

I have been there. This book is for you – with my love.

OUR BACKGROUND

We were fifteen when Jeanne first came on my radar. Both only children of parents who came from large families, we had a lot in common. We were working class, but with aspirations of moving up a notch or two. She was a classy girl. Quite where she acquired her style is a mystery, but she never lost an ounce of it over the years, nor the happy knack of always saying and doing the right thing.

It was 1951, the year of the Festival of Britain. I was besotted with this girl; I took her to be way out of my league – but I got lucky. She responded to my stumbling approach more eagerly than I dared to expect, and agreed to go out with me. It became clear that the attraction was mutual. Almost immediately, we became 'an item', to use the modern expression.

On leaving school, she became a student nurse at the Royal Berkshire Hospital in Reading while I trained as an illustrator and graphic designer with the Home Office. Our mutual attraction survived all the things that can go wrong in a teenage relationship, especially my compulsory service in the Army that took me to North Africa for almost all of the two years. In July 1956, I was home. She was a Staff Nurse on the Male Surgical Ward and loved it – so, I imagine, did her patients.

Two years later we were married. We rented a house in Sunningdale where I picked up my career in the Home Office. Our son Jonathan was born early in 1962 and Jeanne gave up nursing. Later that year a career opportunity for me took us to Faringdon, at the other end of Berkshire, where we were able to afford our first house and where Lizzie came into our world. A subsequent career move brought us to the beautiful Isle of Purbeck in Dorset where Sarah joined the team.

We moved gently up the property ladder, culminating in our much-loved family home 'The Seagull' in Swanage. Twenty years later, when the family were all grown up, Jeanne and I drifted even more gently down, via a thatched cottage in the quaintly named Dorset village of Wool for eight years, a smaller house back in Swanage (where the garden was hewn out of Purbeck stone) to the very comfortable apartment, also in Swanage, where I am writing these words.

In 2008, we celebrated our Golden Wedding Anniversary in style at The Grand Hotel in Swanage, looking across the sea to the Isle of Wight on the sort of day you have no right to expect in an English summer – wall-to-wall sunshine. We could see no reason why we shouldn't do something similar for our Diamond Wedding and were tempted to book the hotel ten years in advance.

We were in good shape for our age and had always taken reasonable care of ourselves. There had been a few health issues that had been a bit worrying at the time but not hugely significant. How very wrong we were . . .

The story that follows is based on extracts from my notebooks and diaries. To help you to make more sense of them I have added subsequent notes in italics.

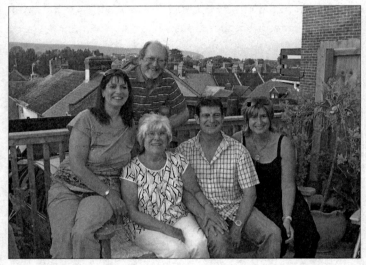

In the family this picture is known as 'The Famous Five'.
Brian is at the back. The front row is: Lizzie, Jeanne,
Jonathan and Sarah.

INTRODUCTIONS

What we would have done without the continual and unconditional support of our family, I cannot imagine.

It may help you if I draw up a cast list.

My name is Brian, the author of this book.

The main character is the lovely Jeanne, the love of my life, who has been at the core of my being since we were fifteen years old.

We have three children; all are in good marriages with children of their own.

As a family unit, we could ask for no more.

Jonathan, our son, is married to Tracey, and they have two sons:

Rick (Richard) and Ben.

Lizzie (Elizabeth), daughter No. 1, is married to Bruce, and they have one son and three daughters:

Luke, Rose, Laura and Annie.

Sarah, daughter No. 2, is married to Paul, and they have one son and one daughter:

Matt (Matthew) and Ems (Emily)

ACKNOWLEDGEMENTS

My deep gratitude to my family is obvious when reading this book. I could not have managed without their love and unconditional support as we picked our way through the horrifying traumas that characterise this little-known disease. But this is no reason not to acknowledge their continuing help during the writing of this book. They have read and re-read the manuscript many times and dredged their more reliable memories to plug the holes in mine.

Without the encouragement of my friend Brian McIvor this book would not have been written. He has powers of persuasion that should come with a health warning. He is probably the only person I know that makes a seemingly ridiculous proposition, like me writing a book, sound perfectly feasible.

Claire Waring, my copy editor, has done a superb job in polishing the text. She has painstakingly ironed out my idiosyncratic use of punctuation and capital letters. Even more importantly she has read the text carefully to ensure uninterrupted narrative flow for the reader. I am very grateful.

Finally, I must thank everyone at York Publishing Services for making the production of this book seem so easy. Every stage of the process has been clearly spelled out; timescales and budgets have been maintained, and there has never been any doubt that the project was in capable hands. Special thanks are due to the Design Manager, Clare Brayshaw, who guided me through every stage of the production.

CHAPTER ONE

Friday 15 November 2013

Just recently Jeanne has become a bit forgetful. Not of
past events: she remembers them in clear-cut detail. It is
picking her way through everyday life where her memory
is letting her down. It's probably just an age thing; part of
her charm has always been a benign, but slightly oblique,
view of the world. It may be nothing but I have an uneasy
feeling that it hasn't to be ignored.

Saturday 16 November 2013

Christmas is approaching and her grip on it seems to be
slipping. She has always loved Christmas and has always
assumed control of the whole palaver: cards, presents,
decorations, the lot. My job is to do as I'm told – and
provide the money.

Yesterday we sat down to make a start on the Christmas
cards. I was nicely relaxed until it became evident that she
was uncertain what to do. Yet we have been using the
system, her system, for a goodish number of years. I don't
understand what is happening.

*She had always been the lead player, selecting the
appropriate card and finding the right page in the
address book. I would write the card, address the
envelope and pass it back to her for checking,
sealing and stamping. It was then recorded in her
'Christmas Book', along with details of the cards
sent to us, ready for reference next year. You can
see, we are talking serious organisation!*

As always, she bought the cards well in advance, but this year the pile doesn't seem big enough. Selecting the appropriate card is troubling her and entering the information into 'The Book' is taking much longer than usual. Very gently, I am easing her through the process, without actually taking over.

The shortfall in cards was accounted for. She put a couple of boxes in a drawer – in the bedroom. I found them quite by chance.

Sunday 17 November 2013

Job done! It was a relief when she said that she couldn't have done it without me. A relief because realising that she is struggling, and relying on my help, is much better than going through life doing batty things without realising it. But what in the world is happening to her?

It seems more than just a memory thing. Early this morning, I sneaked a look in the Christmas Book. I was shocked. The columns are drawn in a wobbly freehand. The writing is recognisably hers and legible – but it's smaller and wandering all over the page. Does she think it looks OK, or does she realise she is struggling with that as well? I'm not sure, but my guess is that she is aware that she has problems, but is doing her best to ignore them. Quite why, I'm not sure: stiff upper-lip probably.

NOTE: Smaller handwriting does have some significance; the lack of neatness on the page is similar. Mention both to your patient's doctor.

As you can imagine, the upshot of all this was a subtle change in our relationship. We had always been equal partners in decision-making; now I was having to take the primary role, but with great subtlety.

Monday 18 November 2013

I woke up in the night thinking about all of this. Her eyesight could be the problem. It makes perfect sense. She was never happy after the second cataract op.

Both her eyes had undergone cataract removal earlier that year. After each procedure, she'd had difficulty in seeing for a few days and the latter one was particularly troublesome with a lot of residual discomfort.

Tuesday 19 November 2013

We talked about her eyesight this afternoon. I was apprehensive but it seemed a kindness now I have a physical rather than a mental cause to account for the difficulties that emerged doing the Christmas cards. She seems relieved at my 'diagnosis' and, on the face of it, seems more relaxed.

Thursday 2 January 2014

That's it! We've survived everything that Christmas and New Year could do to destroy the equal partnership image. Nobody suspects a thing; to everyone that matters we are still Jeanne & Brian, Mum & Dad, Nana & Grandpa. I have been surreptitiously stepping in when anything looks difficult. We can carry on like this indefinitely.

The situation seems nicely under control but I have to be prepared. I believe I can tackle any difficulty if I have the right knowledge. So, I have down-loaded a couple of books on to my Kindle: one on dementia in general and the other on Alzheimer's disease in particular – just in case.

The books were an interesting read but not very reassuring. You will probably find, as I did, that almost all you read will focus on Alzheimer's disease as the worst possible outcome. All other forms of dementia get only a few passing paragraphs, almost as if they are of little consequence.

One piece of very helpful advice emerges from both books. They stress the importance of avoiding conflict. Throughout our life together we have never had problems with holding opposing opinions; now, the silliest things can set us at odds. This afternoon Jeanne said that I'd left the light on in the downstairs cloakroom. I knew this wasn't the case but took the line of least resistance by simply saying sorry. It worked! An hour later she apologised because she had just discovered Harpic in the bowl and knows that she must have done it. Had I contested it the air would have been bluer than the water.

Agreement became my default position. The tricky bit was when I knew that Jeanne was wrong and it might have been dangerous not to correct her. A good example was when she decided her life would take a turn for the better if she started driving again. All we needed to do, she thought, was change our Toyota Yaris for the smaller Toyota Aygo. Clearly, she was no longer capable of driving but this was not the ideal time to say so. It took all my patience and diplomacy over several days to prevent this seemingly minor dispute from turning into a monster.

NOTE: If you are faced with this sort of dilemma I implore you please don't yield to temptation. Please don't say, "Don't be ridiculous!"

My solution was to say that I had heard that a new model of Aygo, with a fully automatic gearbox that would be ideal for, her was due for release this year.

I said that I had spoken to the dealers – and they were expecting it to be available in September. She never mentioned it again.

Friday 3 January 2014

The short-term memory seems to be getting worse. Surreptitious reading on Kindle suggests that Jeanne's condition would be classed as a 'mild cognitive impairment' or MCI, as they call it in the trade. Treatment is not necessary: if diagnosed, the patient becomes part of a 'watch and wait' procedure. I don't think consulting our GP has any value at the moment: I can watch and wait at least as well as he can.

Medics use acronyms a lot. This is hardly surprising given the long, multi-syllable words that are part of their everyday vocabulary. I will follow that convention but will elaborate on them where necessary.

Friday 31 January 2014

The MCI doesn't seem any worse and we've been on a nicely even keel for most of the month. We have been shopping in Poole at least once a week, followed by lunch out. She likes this. And there have been some nice evening meals with various parts of our family. It is still that time of year, when reasons to celebrate abound.

Things seem very much back to normal. I've even found a few hours to do a line and wash drawing of one of Swanage's more attractive houses.

Friday 21 February 2014

The relaxed state has been maintained. We have celebrated both our birthdays with as many of the family that could make it.

Jeanne continues to have some bother with her eyes. It's less about her vision: more about general discomfort and itching. I'm bathing them for her every morning and have spoken to the Eye Unit at Bournemouth Hospital on the basis that it is probably a residual effect from the cataract procedures. They think that this is unlikely and have recommended an 'over-the-counter' eye-drop to alleviate dryness.

Tuesday 4 March 2014

This afternoon I called the Eye Unit again and spoke to a different nurse practitioner. I explained Jeanne's symptoms and immediately she said that it sounds like blepharitis, a condition of high nuisance value but harmless. It is controlled by good eye hygiene involving warm compresses, gentle massage and bathing.

You will realise I'm sure that the condition was incidental to the cognitive impairment, but there were two important connections.

a) The MCI made it difficult for her to remember the order of the stages of treatment.

b) The treatment highlighted a new difficulty: Jeanne was losing her spatial awareness. This made the whole process a hit and miss affair, with the latter being more likely.

I had to be involved; it became an extension to my role as her carer and added the best part of half-an-hour to the getting-up procedure, in which I was also involved.

NOTE: If you feel that someone you are caring for is losing their spatial awareness, you should tell your doctor. It does have diagnostic significance.

Wednesday 19 March 2014

We have a new obstacle: her mobile phone. Sending and receiving text messages is giving her grief. A few weeks ago, she began asking me to read the incoming messages, and to check her outgoing messages were OK. Shortly after, I was entering the text for her. Now I'm doing the whole thing: compiling the message, entering the text and reading it back to her before sending. It's time consuming – but nobody suspects a thing. Lizzie got her 'Happy Birthday' text today, and assumes it's from her Mum – rather than her Mum's 'secretary'!

Jeanne has always been capable in managing her medication; now she is uncertain of the purpose of each tablet, when to take it and when to re-order. I've tried to help by buying her a box to set out her pills for the week: one compartment for each day. But she doesn't like it and says it is confusing – probably because she is no longer sure which day of the week we're on. It is another thing to worry about – and another thing for me to do.

It is probably obvious to you by now that I was beginning to entertain doubts about the credibility of my earlier 'inadequate eyesight' theory.

Sunday 23 March 2014

Short-term memory is the real problem. As I see it, the short-term memory provides all the links in normal thinking and reasoning. I've persuaded her we have to deal with the deficiency as a couple and accept it as a disability. No one else needs to know; it can be 'our little secret'. She is trying to replace the missing links by writing notes in her diary.

NOTE: It is hugely important to boost the patient's confidence at every available opportunity. I reminded

Jeanne repeatedly that it was only her short-term memory that was letting her down and that her memory of past events was way above average – and a lot better than mine. She was also very good at remembering directions when we were in the car and had tremendous command of all the shortcuts through Bournemouth and Poole.

Minutes later she decided to make a note of her main problem in her diary. But she had already forgotten what it was called . . .

Saturday 29 March 2014

Caring for her is becoming a full-time job, but we are still getting out and about. We seemed to manage 'our little secret' just fine when we went with the whole family to Center Parcs recently, to celebrate Lizzie's fiftieth birthday.

Nobody knew that I had to do most of the packing for Jeanne and help her decide what she needed to take. She managed very well during the time we were there. No one suspected a thing.

Last night we had Jonathan and Tracey for a meal. I've been cooking since I retired twenty years ago so no cover-ups were necessary. It was a lovely evening.

CHAPTER TWO

Tuesday 1 April 2014

Jeanne's favourite way of spending a day is still going shopping and having lunch out. Her taste in clothes is becoming less self-assured and she doesn't like trying things on in the shops. The intricate fixings of women's clothes can be tricky without my help, and she doesn't want the shop assistant to know about that. So, we buy the clothes, try them on at home and, more often than not, take them back the next day. Sometimes we re-purchase them the day after that. I don't mind; she is happy.

She still had a full set of credit and debit cards but the chance of her remembering the pin numbers was becoming remote. She was very happy to take the soft option of letting me pay. I used to say to the family: "Mum is like the Queen: she doesn't carry money," and then as an afterthought, "but she has a better dress sense!"

Deciding what she wants to eat for lunch can also be a bit of a challenge, so she tends always to have the same thing or to ask me to choose for her.

There is no huge significance in this but it is worth drawing your attention to the possibility. Once I became aware of the difficulty, I tried to make it easy by drawing her attention to anything on the menu that would appeal to her.

But she was still lovely company and we enjoyed our meals out, as long as it was just the two of us. That included the family who at that time, as far as we were aware, suspected nothing.

NOTE: That she had started worrying that other people might find out was curiously reassuring. From my reading, this isn't a typical worry of Alzheimer's patients: they are more likely to recede into a closed world of her own, in which they become increasingly unaware of other peoples' identities.

Wednesday 16 April 2014

Yesterday we went to John Lewis where an ill-designed tray stand, at the entrance to the cafeteria, was lying in wait for her. The ensuing collision removed a piece of shin about the size of a pound coin which was unlikely to stop bleeding without some sort of dressing. The store first-aider fell upon us; the result was secure enough to get us home – but only just. We made a rather better job of it when we got home but it seemed advisable to seek professional help from the Minor Injuries Unit at Swanage Hospital. A nurse cleaned the wound properly, dressed it expertly and suggested he saw us again in four days.

Throughout all this, Jeanne was completely her old self. It was almost as though being in a hospital environment had taken her back through the years, to the world of sterile dressings she could understand and which, of course, was almost like living in the past – where her memory was still intact.

Sunday 20 April 2014

Back to Swanage Hospital as instructed. A different nurse said there was no infection; he cleaned it up again, re-dressed it and discharged us.

Once again, she slipped back into 'State Registered Nurse, mode. I wondered if this would always happen in a hospital environment.

Thursday 15 May 2014

We went, with Sarah and Ems, to see the Birmingham Royal Ballet in Poole last night. Jeanne loved every minute of it and, although her mobility has become affected, she walked happily and quite quickly from the car park to the theatre and back; everything seemed completely normal, and perfect.

> NOTE: *It was typical of her condition that behaviour and ability to comprehend was variable – and random, not just from day to day, but by the hour – sometimes by the minute.*
>
> *I don't think she was aware of this characteristic: her deficient short-term memory was failing to supply the links from one moment to the next.*
>
> *What it would mean to you as a carer is that there is a constant need to adjust your responses to match the mental state of the patient. The tricky bit is that other people know nothing of the problem, nor the need to make adjustments.*
>
> *To avoid potential difficulties, I found myself controlling interfaces with other people, but without making it obvious. You will find the need for continual awareness can become very stressful.*

Friday 16 May 2014

The MCI notion, to which the optimist in me still clings, is beginning to lose its validity. The realist is thinking that Jeanne may well be suffering from some sort of dementia, but not yet severe enough to consult our GP.

My reading at that time described several types and levels of dementia. Needless to say, I was still grasping at one of the milder categories. This was supported by the fact that a lot of what I was seeing still didn't seem typical of the onset of the dreaded Alzheimer's disease.

Tuesday 20 May 2014

As long as we are alone she's fine, but a bit wobbly with anyone else, even close relatives – by which I mean our children and grandchildren. But, as the weather improves and the evenings get longer, invitations to barbecues and garden parties will threaten.

I used the word 'threaten' very deliberately. To her, who had always been able to slip into party mood at the drop of a hat, the thought of socialising was becoming a very real threat – to 'our little secret'.

Later that day

A new problem has emerged of which I can make neither head nor tail. From time to time she seems to withdraw into herself in a way I can't understand. It is hard to describe, but I have to try. Her face freezes into one position, as though her nervous system has shut down. It lasts for only a few minutes and is best dealt with by sitting quietly until she 'comes back'. I haven't mentioned it to her; I wouldn't know how to start. I hope it is 'just one of those things', a passing phase perhaps. In my mind, she goes into 'sphinx mode'.

For several reasons, my guiding principle was not to say or do anything that would indicate that the little oddities were at all obvious. Keeping her placid was fundamental to maintaining her peace of mind – and mine.

Wednesday 28 May 2014

We should have been at the Conservative Club for Quiz Night. Mercifully, she has developed some sort of bug and really isn't well enough to go. What a relief!

We both greeted this genuine excuse to cancel a threatening social occasion with enthusiasm. For Jeanne, fear of making a fool of herself was very, very real. For me, dreaming up plausible excuses became more and more taxing.

Sunday 1 June 2014

Now I've caught the same bug and feel dreadful. We should have been in Daventry this weekend with Lizzie and Bruce, but I had to call it off. When I phoned Lizzie, she was very understanding and seemed almost relieved. She said that she had been wondering if we were well enough for the journey anyway. This has set me thinking. Is she beginning to suspect something?

Thursday 12 June 2014

It is Paul's fiftieth birthday party at Middle Beach Café on Saturday. Jeanne hasn't said anything but I am worrying how she is going to cope with it.

The Café is Paul's own business so I knew she would be familiar with the venue but, additional to our family, there were going to be people there we knew less well. That was likely to be a bit of a challenge for her.

If only our children knew of her difficulties, they would be able to help shield her from any embarrassing moments.

> NOTE: *It was very tempting to talk to them, but I was ever mindful of 'our little secret'. Now I can see the position I had adopted was wrong and I'm not sure why I persisted with it. Almost certainly I was in denial to a certain extent; probably it was out of loyalty to Jeanne; and I guess I didn't want to worry Jonathan, Lizzie and Sarah. Some of this may seem admirable. In truth it was stupid!*
>
> *My firm advice to you is: seek all the help you can get – as soon as possible.*

Monday 16 June 2014

The birthday party was a wonderful evening. Jeanne survived it without embarrassment. I kept close by to ease her through any conversations that could have given her problems. She seemed happy and relaxed.

Wednesday 25 June 2014

Jeanne is beginning to deteriorate physically: in particular, her movements are becoming stilted and her sense of balance is not reliable. Her ability to manage the stairs in the house and the steps in the garden is beginning to worry me.

> *Our garden was on four different levels, built from Purbeck stone and fraught with the hazards of uneven steps and jagged edges. Just getting in to the house through the back door was threatening, even for the able-bodied.*

This morning I introduced the subject of a possible move to test her reaction. She seems to like the idea of single-level accommodation but I imagine that she thinks it will be a bungalow. A flat would be a better option: I have more than enough to do without having to look after a garden.

Saturday 28 June 2014

That was a surprise. She likes the idea of a flat and reminded me that, when we were at the cottage in Wool, she always said that when we returned to Swanage she liked the idea of living in one of the flats in the centre of town. Bungalows don't seem to be part of her thinking, so – the search begins.

I didn't realise at the time what an important difference this was going to make. It added a new focus to our life; it gave us something to concentrate on together that didn't depend on her memory, nor on her diminishing ability to organise. Best of all there was no tearing hurry: a nice relaxing pastime.

Saturday 5 July 2014

The local paper arrived yesterday and Jeanne had it open to the estate agency pages almost before it hit the doormat! She is enthusiastic for the move and is enjoying having a project to concentrate on.

Swanage Carnival was only a few weeks away. It was an established tradition that our family always gathered in Swanage at that time so, unless anything unmissable cropped up, we decided not to approach the estate agents until it was all over.

Saturday 12 July 2014

Today is our fifty-sixth wedding anniversary. Luke is staying with us for a couple of nights. Although he is now a qualified doctor, he doesn't start his first job until the beginning of August and wants to catch up with some of his old mates in Swanage.

With Luke arriving, family visiting, and meals out, the anniversary was hectic. Jeanne coped with it all very well, leaving me quietly optimistic.

Saturday 19 July 2014

Some invitations are easy to wriggle out of but, during carnival week, almost every evening there is 'something on'. Some of them will be close family only and she should be OK; it is the ones with a wider spread of guests that make me feel apprehensive about Jeanne's fear of socialising.

Monday 21 July 2014

A new threat has just cropped up: we have been asked if, during carnival week, we can accommodate our granddaughter Laura and her partner Scott, with their little boy Zachary – our first great-grandchild. In the normal way, we would have been delighted, but we are a long way from normality. How Jeanne will cope with sharing the house with a whole family, albeit small, has put my mind in a complete whirl. Help!!!

This was another occasion when I should have shared her problem with the family. Why was I so determined to maintain the secrecy? Sheer cussedness probably. Absolutely ridiculous.

The reason it cropped up? Since their most recent visit to Swanage, ours is the only house without a dog and, as Zachary is not used to dogs, it seemed a sensible option.

Tuesday 22 July 2014

I've talked it through with Jeanne, as best I can. She doesn't fully understand the subtleties of my worries but would far rather they stayed with us than allow the extent of her problems to become common knowledge.

Saturday 26 July 2014

They arrived in time to go and see the carnival fireworks. We are staying at home and making the most of having the house to ourselves.

CHAPTER THREE

Tuesday 29 July 2014

This morning Jeanne went to Middle Beach Café with the girls. I rushed round the house cleaning as best I could and then made the most of my time by doing some preparatory drawings on the beach where the fishermen park their boats, lobster pots and nets. I'm preparing for a picture requested by Luke for his birthday.

We are due at Sarah's house for a buffet this evening to which various other people have been invited. Jeanne really doesn't want to go, but I have managed to persuade her that we should just put in an appearance and the minute she wants to leave, just tip me the wink.

Wednesday 30 July 2014

Nobody would have suspected a thing: she was just Jeanne, as usual. A little quiet perhaps but then she has never been a 'mouth-almighty' – far from it. Like I've said before, pure class.

Tonight is barbecue night at Jonathan's and it is likely that there will be more guests that she knows less well, or not at all. I thought for much of the day that a contrived excuse might become necessary but, on the strength of her success last night, I've persuaded her to go. She's none too happy. I've agreed to extricate her the minute she indicates she's ready to leave. I shall say that I am feeling out of sorts. Fingers crossed she makes it.

Thursday 31 July 2014

She was anxious all day but, come the evening, she managed perfectly well again: we stayed for long enough and she seemed normal enough to allay any suspicions. She actually left my side at one point and sat outside with the girls while I talked in the summer house with the chaps. Another worry evaporates.

Tomorrow is a stay at home day; no garden parties are planned. The family will go to the funfair on 'the rec'. We will be allowed, expected probably, to stay at home. What a relief!

Friday 1 August 2014

I was up soon after sunrise today and it is still only a little after the crack of dawn. The weather is good. Once our breakfast is over and Jeanne is ready to start the day, I can prune the clematis before our guests are up and about. There is a good chance I shall finish it today, whilst the gang sample the delights of Swanage at Carnival time, and we can relax in the garden and not worry about a thing.

Much later the same day

Why did I tempt providence by writing that? I was several feet up on the decking, pruning the clematis, when Jeanne called me from the back door. Whether I tripped, slipped or whether my right leg gave out, or all three, is not clear; suddenly I was hurtling head first towards the paved area below. Split-second thoughts raced through my head. This is going to hurt! The injuries will be serious! I might die! Who is going to look after Jeanne? They are going to have to know!

Somehow, I managed to twist in the air and took the first impact on my shoulder. Then my head whacked into the solid Purbeck paving stones!

The shock and the pain were about equal and I thought I was done for. Then, after a few hazy moments, and against all odds, I realised that I was conscious and, in spite of the pain, everything seemed to be working. Jeanne saw it happening but had no idea what to do. She called Laura, who has neither skills nor experience in first aid – but had the sense to telephone her Mum, Lizzie, who was at Sarah's house. Within minutes I was surrounded by almost the whole family who, as usual, arrived mob-handed – any excuse for a party!

Somebody had dialled 999. The paramedic was in front of me minutes later. He was quick but thorough. He said I was lucky. In a fall like that he would have expected several broken bones as a minimum – but I had got away with it. Normally he would have taken me to A&E at Poole Hospital but, as there was substantial family support, he decided to leave them to call 999 again if I got any worse.

Saturday 2 August 2014

Everything has changed! The fall yesterday started a chain reaction. This morning, my head was sore but, more worryingly, it started spinning every time I moved. Lizzie and Sarah took me to the Minor Injuries Unit at our small local hospital.

Maybe it was the bang on the head that weakened my resolve. Maybe, at last, I was seeing the stupidity of my position. I had to level with them.

"Have you noticed Mum isn't quite herself lately?"

At which point we were called. The Nurse Practitioner re-assured us that my symptoms were consistent with recovery from a severe blow to the head, and that 'there was nothing to worry about'.

Those last few words resonated with us. There most certainly was something for us to worry about, but nothing to do with my fall. There was a lot to talk about.

I was no longer alone with my problems and they were able to talk to me openly about their Mum. We sat outside the hospital for long enough to go through the basic issues. The girls, I think, shed the odd tear; I just about managed not to, but I remember saying that the future looked bleak.

They had been talking to each other a lot, and to Jonathan, who at that time, was perhaps slightly more optimistic. Until recently, all three had taken the view that things couldn't be too bad – because she was still texting them!

Something new has also been bothering them. At Jonathan's barbecue, when Jeanne had left me to join the girls, she had gone into 'sphinx mode', which worried the life out of them. They'd asked her if she was OK but she seemed unaware that anything untoward had happened. They had wondered if they should talk to me about it but decided not to worry me.

There was little else that I could do other than say that from this point on I would keep them fully informed. I told them that if my text messages had two sets of three kisses at the end it was from their Mum and me; if there was only one set it was from me alone, and would probably be about their Mum.

NOTE: The relief of having them in the picture was huge and I now feel qualified to give you emphatic advice. If you find yourself in a similar position tell those nearest to you at the earliest opportunity.

My concept of 'our little secret' was well-meant, but pointless – and stupid!

Sunday 3 August 2014

Earlier today I got a text message from Lizzie. She has been talking to Luke: his professional opinion is that, given her history, the very first thing that should be checked is Jeanne's thyroid function. Cognitive impairment is a recognised sign of an underactive thyroid, particularly in elderly people.

Early in 2013 Jeanne had been given radioiodine treatment for an overactive thyroid. When he discharged her back to our GP, the consultant stipulated that because an underactive thyroid is a possible side effect, her thyroid function should be checked at three months and again at nine months.

This could account for everything. I've just looked into her medical records. It is there – just what I wanted to see. The first test was done but the second test has been missed; she hasn't had a TFT for fourteen months.

TFT: Thyroid Function Test. A sample of blood is taken to measure hormone levels.

Monday 4 August 2014

I can't talk to our GP until 15 August, but it will give me time to discuss the thyroid issue with Jeanne, which means that she has to know that the family knows about 'our little secret'. I think it needs to be done tonight. I am dreading it.

Tuesday 5 August 2014

She didn't take it very well: to be honest the initial reaction was better described as an eruption. I managed to stay calm: it was imperative that I should for the well-being of both of us. I explained why it had been necessary to let our children into the secret – and to assure her that there was no one else in the loop. Later, Sarah got both barrels. Jeanne demanded to know exactly what she was doing that made us all think she wasn't herself.

> NOTE: *Jeanne's anger was uncharacteristic of the level-headed and reasonable woman I had known for more than sixty years. It has to be included as a symptom of her evolving condition.*

> *Eventually she accepted that, if her problems were due to an underactive thyroid, a daily dose of thyroxine would bring the levels up to normal and her short-term memory symptoms would improve rapidly. The clincher was that she had never been happy about the radioactive treatment: this would prove she had been right.*

Friday 15 August 2014

The phone call to the GP achieved what I wanted. He agreed Jeanne's symptoms were typical of an under-active thyroid and apologised for the oversight. He did the paper work for the TFT while he was talking to me.

An appointment has been made for the blood sample to be taken on Monday morning, and the GP will call us on the following afternoon with the result.

> *Although Jeanne was not happy initially, she admitted that she felt much safer with a doctor being involved. I could scarcely wait for the GP's call which I was convinced would lead to the end of all our problems.*

Tuesday 19 August 2014

The thyroid function is down, but not enough to need treating – a disappointment, but not a disaster.

The doctor and Jeanne both thought this result was good. Jeanne is naively interpreting the result as meaning there's nothing wrong with her; quite why the doctor was so cheery he didn't say. There is nothing to cling to now, apart from the GP saying that he will repeat the TFT in three months.

Wednesday 20 August 2014

I am no longer alone. Knowing the family is available when the going gets tough is comforting, but this afternoon I tried to work on the drawing for Luke's birthday, but without much success. I can't concentrate. My duty of care occupies most of my thinking.

Monday 25 August 2014

Sarah dropped in for coffee and a chat today. It is easier for me now that she, Lizzie and Jonathan understand the situation. I suspect it would be easier for Jeanne if only I could persuade her that the age-old stigma about mental health problems is no longer valid. The trouble is that she knows as well as I do that a lot of people still talk about it in whispers.

'Alzheimer's' is the dreaded word. My reading suggests that it is the worst possible outcome, and that none of the other causes of dementia are as threatening. Could stress be a possible cause? Am I clutching at another straw?

It is unlikely to be the only cause, but worry about how she would manage if I become incapacitated, or if I should die, occupies a lot of her thinking. Given our advancing years, the stress level could be part of the problem.

I think now that I was muddling the cause and effect. It seems much more likely that she realised that her mental faculties were going into recession, and that was the main reason for her worrying about how she would cope without me.

Thursday 28 August 2014

I ran all this past her last night and she admitted that she had felt vulnerable for months, but made no attempt to associate this with her cognitive impairment.

I was still expecting the impairment to be transitory and could not accept that Jeanne might be in serious trouble. Online I found evidence of research being done on the possibility of stress leading to MCI, but I could find no published results. Further investigation suggested that MCI could progress to dementia as a result of stress. But nothing was found to support the possibility that removing stress from a MCI could reverse the process.

Monday 31 August 2014

Jeanne's school-friend Doreen has arrived to spend a day or two with us, as she does from time to time. Because we know her well I don't anticipate any problems.

Wednesday 3 September 2014

I was right. Everything was nicely relaxed and Doreen has gone home to Devon, not suspecting a thing; or if she does, she is keeping it to herself.

Monday 8 September 2014

My optimism had a welcome boost over the weekend: Jeanne decided to make some rock buns, something she hasn't done for a year or two. She needed a little help with weighing up the ingredients but this was no surprise. In the days when she did all the cooking, she always used to believe that accurate measurement was over-rated. She preferred working by touch, feel and finger-dipping. She no longer has that confidence – but the rock buns were excellent.

NOTE: Once again, it seemed as though we might have turned a corner. I should have known better: it was just another good day amongst the many 'up-and-down' days, none of which is in any way predictable.

Wednesday 10 September 2014

Jeanne continues to worry about how she will manage if I suddenly become ill, or die. If she needs urgent help how will she get it? She has lost the ability to cope with medical issues. She has lost the ability use her mobile phone for texting – and she is uncertain how to use it to call anyone.

Her worry was understandable, and dated back to 1 January 2012, when I had a nocturnal seizure in which I lost consciousness. Still perfectly capable at that time, Jeanne started my resuscitation then rang Sarah for support. Sarah dialled 999 on her way to us. I woke up looking into the bearded face of a paramedic. Off I went to A&E where it was decided to treat me as an outpatient.

Subsequently, all manner of tests over several months showed nothing abnormal. In August 2012, the same thing happened. This time I was admitted to hospital and a 24/7 ECG showed that sometimes my heart-rate dropped unacceptably low, so a pacemaker was installed. There have been no further seizures, but you can see why she was worried.

A couple of days ago, I dropped in to my usual phone supplier to see if they had a very simple phone that even Jeanne could manage. They came up with what appeared to be the ideal solution, so I bought one.

Much like the mobile phones of a few years ago, it has a numerical keyboard, plus three extra keys labelled A, B and C under which can be stored three specific numbers. Perfect! Press A for Jonathan, B for Lizzie or C for Sarah, followed by a GREEN call button – and it doesn't really matter which one she calls. Can she manage it? No way! At the moment, she is blaming the stupid phone!

NOTE: You need to be ready for this reaction. Dealing with it demands huge reserves of patience and you have to be prepared to fail. I persevered for several days and, by writing very simple instructions for her, she eventually achieved something approaching a 50% success rate. How long she remembers how to do it is by no means certain. It is all very taxing.

CHAPTER FOUR

Monday 15 September 2014

We have started looking for a suitable flat to be our new home. There are one or two possibilities but we need a valuation for this house to fix a budget price.

It was time to speak to our friendly family of estate agents whom we had known since 1978, when they found us our beloved family home, 'The Seagull'.

A small breakthrough on the texting front yesterday: Sarah came to do her Mum's hair and after she had gone Jeanne managed to send her a 'thank you' text – more or less single-handed. All I did was to check she was sending it to the right number because she was wary of sending it to the wrong person. This concern was encouraging because I felt it wasn't typical of someone suffering from dementia.

This, of course, was another good example of the fluctuating nature of her condition: just because she managed to do a text message yesterday doesn't mean she could do it today. But her concern at the possibility of sending it to the wrong person seemed to be consistent.

Sunday 21 September 2014

The thought of moving is exciting and looking at property an interesting pastime, but deep down I am anguishing about Jeanne. Am I doing all the right things to keep her happy and secure? Tomorrow the agents are coming to value the house.

Monday 22 September 2014

The agents' valuation is much as expected. Now we can start looking around seriously. Ideally, it should be a short level walk from the town centre and not at the top of one of the steepest hills in Swanage, as we are at the moment. By the same token, it should either be on the ground floor or accessible by a good and reliable lift. The other issue is adequate car parking space for us and visitors.

Moving to an apartment will be a massive change in our circumstances and it might be difficult for her, but it will make it so much easier for me to do my job, which is to care for the girl I fell in love with when we were teenagers.

Nothing had changed in the way I felt about Jeanne but it was a job from which there was very little respite. Deep down, hidden from view by my outward optimism, I was realising that it could only get worse. My hopes were now pinned on the next TFT scheduled for 5 November. The underactive thyroid notion made so much sense, and a prescription for thyroxine tablets would put an end to my constant agonising.

Thursday 25 September 2014

We have looked at two flats. The first matched most of our requirements: it seemed in good condition and had the right number of rooms; the lift and car park were adequate but the building looked a bit run down. The second just didn't seem right.

Wednesday 1 October 2014

Earlier today we took Sarah and Paul with us to have another look at the first flat. They agreed on the state of the building and Paul noticed that one corner of the building needed re-pointing. I have turned it down.

The agents have nothing else at the moment, Apparently, there is usually a lull at this time of year, so I have put the potential move on hold until the spring.

This also bought me some thinking time. Where might the cognitive impairment be heading? If it should prove to be Alzheimer's disease would a move of that magnitude be the best thing for her? Would she be able to adjust to a different environment? By the spring we should be better informed.

Thursday 9 October 2014

Last weekend we got away to Daventry for a few days: for me it was a bit of relaxation, once we got there. Getting ready to go was far from relaxing. The truth is that Jeanne can no longer organise herself. I had to decide what to take for her: clothes, medications, toiletries, hot brush – you name it.

After Lizzie and Bruce had gone to work on Monday I asked her if she fancied a little shopping trip to Banbury which is about ten miles away. You bet she did! About halfway there she suddenly said:

"You're going the wrong way!"

I knew we weren't: I was following the signs carefully. A few minutes later she said she was certain that I had gone wrong somewhere. The signs took us to the town centre and I parked up. Suddenly she said:

"This is Banbury! I thought we were going to Rugby!"

Interesting. Her long-term memory knew the way to both Banbury and Rugby but her short-term memory had forgotten where we were going.

Friday 10 October 2014

We're home now. Last weekend in Daventry I said we would look after Luke's cat, Anastasia. Lizzie is bringing her tomorrow. Surprisingly, Jeanne isn't very enthusiastic. We've had a lot of cats and she loved and cared for them all without exception. My idea is that another one will help to give her a new focus.

Luke inherited the cat when he was a medical student. When he qualified, he brought the cat home with him, for his sister, Laura, to look after. Unfortunately, she already had a cat and the two didn't get on. Even worse, Anastasia was terrified of Zachary.

Saturday 11 October 2014

Lizzie arrived just before lunch with Anastasia. It seems so right to have a cat in the house again, but this one is a very frightened little thing.

Sunday 12 October 2014

The cat is a bit of a puzzle. She's around early morning but at around eight am she disappears without trace. She has never been an outdoor cat so we know she's somewhere in the house. Then, about five pm, she re-appears and stays around most of the evening.

Friday 17 October 2014

I've solved the cat's daily disappearing trick. She has discovered a small space underneath Jeanne's armchair hidden by a flap of leather. The space is just right for her to wriggle in, to curl up in and feel safe. Even more interesting is the reason why. She disappears at the time she is used to Zachary getting up at Laura's – and she comes out at his bedtime.

The bigger conundrum, for which there seemed to be no solution, was against all expectations: Jeanne wasn't taking to her at all, neither was she in the least interested in looking after her. I had given myself one more thing to do.

NOTE: This episode pointed up a personality change that no one would have expected. For the greater part of her life, Jeanne was unable to resist any animal.

Saturday 18 October 2015

My cousin Janie, and her husband Geoff, are coming to Bournemouth next weekend to celebrate their wedding anniversary. Several weeks ago, we arranged to meet them for lunch. Now I have a problem: Jeanne feels quite unable to fulfil this engagement. She has known Janie as long as she has known me, indeed Janie was her bridesmaid, and they are the easiest people in the world to get along with.

There was only one solution; I had to say that Jeanne had a bug and was unwell. Janie accepted this without question, but I felt my negotiating skills were a bit below par and it all sounded a bit hollow.

Recently Jeanne has complained of occasional dizzy spells. I think she is rather frightened by them. Just another little thing to add to the worry list.

Tuesday 28 October 2104

Yesterday we bought a new vacuum cleaner. Jeanne has been pretty much the sole user of the one we have had for many years. It still works but it is too heavy for her now, and is a very real threat when she uses it on the stairs. The new one is a lightweight rechargeable model which would be so much easier for her – if only she could learn how to use it. The short-term memory difficulty makes it impossible for her to learn anything new. I like to think of myself as a patient man and I am trying to teach her just one thing a day.

> *NOTE: Great idea in theory! In practice of no value at all. Quite simply, to learn one thing a day it is necessary to remember from one minute to the next – Jeanne can't.*
>
> *I thought it was just modern technology that she was struggling with, but it is anything new. I now do the vacuuming!*

Sunday 2 November 2014

Earlier today, Jeanne wanted to save me a job by using the old vacuum cleaner but, because of its weight and her frailty, I had to be with her all the time. The threat of her tripping over the power lead makes it impossible. Vacuuming has to be my job – but at least the new lightweight cleaner makes it easier.

Wednesday 5 November 2014

This morning we went to the phlebotomist to give the sample for her next TFT. We are due to see the GP six days from now.

Saturday 8 November 2015

We had a little shopping trip to Poole two days ago: today we are off again to return the fleece she bought.

On the way back, we bought an assortment of cat food: I tried to interest Jeanne in choosing what Anastasia might like. No interest whatsoever.

When we got home, her only interest in the cat was completely illogical. She began to worry that Anastasia might get out of the house, by wriggling through the letter box! Anastasia is a fully grown adult cat. The letterbox was normal size and had a spring-loaded draught excluder which the postman struggled to push letters through. For the cat to get out was not just unlikely – it was a physical impossibility. Jeanne took my opinion as clear evidence that I didn't share her understanding of how clever cats are. Later on, she tried running the problem past both Lizzie and Sarah but could convince neither of them. She was very cross!

Tuesday 11 November 2014

We saw the GP today. Big relief: Jeanne's thyroid levels have dropped. Start on 50mg daily of thyroxine for 28 days, increasing to 100mg daily. I have high hopes.

He also asked her a few random questions based on the Mini Mental State Examination (MMSE). She was OK on some, on others not so good. She could spell WORLD backwards and give the months of the year backwards; but she wasn't at all sure what day of the week we were on, nor the date.

He asked us if we have heard of the 'Memory Gateway'. We haven't. It is a relatively new set-up which may be the sort of help we are looking for, but he had little experience to tell us about. I must do some work on this.

NOTE: MMSE is a test widely used by doctors to give a quick assessment of a patient's mental state. Jeanne wasn't happy about it; she felt the questions were exposing her to ridicule.

NOTE: The 'Memory Gateway' is a route for patients to access the Dorset Memory Assessment Service, a joint operation between Dorset Healthcare (NHS) and the Alzheimer's Society that leads, eventually, to a full assessment by a psychiatrist.

It seemed worth further investigation. You may have something similar in your area.

Friday 14 November 2014

After only one dose of thyroxine, Jeanne seems a little more switched on. Last night we went to a concert in Poole by the John Wilson Orchestra for which we paid £45 each. I asked her what she thought of it. She thought it was OK but expected more for the cost of the tickets.

I recorded this because, as an example of her thinking, it is not typical. Indeed, what is typical? This shows how her state of mind alters from day to day. She would have made this judgement a couple of years ago, when her mind was still all of a piece.

Monday 17 November 2014

The new thyroxine tablets are identical to her bendroflumethiazide tablets: they are the same small size and white with a C in a circle on one side and something too small to read on the other. She is on 'tablet strike' until I sort it out with the pharmacist.

With a magnifying glass, the pharmacist was able to show me that the thyroxine could be identified by T/A in a circle on the reverse side. The bendroflumethiazide had B/A in a similar position. I wonder what genius allowed that to happen? It was just one more thing that I needed to supervise to ensure she didn't take two of one tablet and none of the other.

Wednesday 19 November 2014

I have been looking at the Memory Gateway website. It looks promising. Once we are referred, an assessor visits us at home to establish how we are managing with everyday life.

A specialist nurse follows up a week or two later to make a thorough mental assessment and report back to the team psychiatrist. The psychiatrist makes a diagnosis, advises on the appropriate care pathway and sets up a support network to enable the patient to live as normal a life as possible.

It is worth a try. Jeanne seems OK with it but, since the MMSE episode, she seems threatened by anything that puts her under the microscope.

CHAPTER FIVE

Saturday 22 November 2014

Yesterday Jeanne was a bit out of sorts. Sarah and I had each had a 'bug' during the week so I think it had caught up with her. She stayed in bed until mid-morning and, as a result, forgot her meds. I was busy filing my tax return online and didn't discover the omission until late evening.

She was still using the seven-compartment box, with each compartment labelled with a day of the week but, as emerged at the recent GP visit, she often didn't know what day of the week it is, so she had waited to ask me – but forgot. You will find this sort of thing, though trivial, can make unreasonable claims on the patience.

Monday 24 November 2014

This morning I booked the next TFT for 30 December. In the meantime, we have to get through Christmas. Her reaction to social events is still unpredictable. She used to look forward to them; now they represent a threat. I feel anxious for her.

The thyroxine may have been improving some elements of her thyroid function, such as her awareness of what was going on, but overall, her cognitive impairment seemed to be worsening.

Getting herself up and dressed takes ages. Yet when she appears downstairs she will often say that she hasn't done her hair yet, or hasn't cleaned her teeth.

She knows that today is Monday – or is that just a lucky guess!

Sunday 30 November 2014

It's time to start the Christmas cards again! It was this job last year that ignited my suspicion that things were going a bit haywire. At least I am prepared now.

A bigger problem would have been Christmas presents for the family but Jonathan, Lizzie and Sarah have advised me that gift vouchers will be perfectly acceptable.

That was a huge relief because I could buy vouchers in a couple of shops in Swanage. But even vouchers had to be wrapped and made to look appropriately 'Christmassy'. Jeanne wanted to be involved. It slowed the process down, but it was necessary to encourage her as much as possible even though time was at a premium.

Monday 1 December 2014

I am struggling at the moment with cooking: I still want to do good healthy food using fresh ingredients, but time is against me. I have to face it – I am a full-time carer, with an emphasis on 'full-time'.

NOTE: By this time, it should have been obvious that engaging the help of a care agency was inevitable. I was reluctant to accept this. Take my advice: accept that caring is an all-consuming life-changer. By 'carrying on as usual' you are putting yourself at risk. Financial help is available in the UK. Apply to the Department of Work and Pensions (DWP) for the Attendance Allowance as soon as possible.

Wednesday 3 December 2014

Now I have a cold and feel absolutely wretched. It's bad enough getting a cold as Christmas approaches at normal times – but this one is far from normal.

Thursday 11 December 2014

That's it! All the cards and presents that need to be posted are away and I've renewed the car insurance. What next?

Traditionally we had exchanged small, but actual, presents with one or two friends. Jeanne wanted to keep up the tradition mainly because if we stopped they might suspect something. Unfortunately, by tradition the values are too small to substitute vouchers. That was all I needed! I know the problem was solved; I can't remember how. But I made up my mind to fix this problem before next year.

Thursday 18 December 2014

I think we are almost prepared for Christmas now. I am nearly exhausted and once or twice I have been close to losing my sense of humour.

We have been into Poole at least three times for no good reason. The most recent was to a shop where Jeanne had seen a dressing gown she'd liked the previous day. The shop doesn't sell dressing gowns. On another day, she decided there was a need to return a pair of trousers: when we got there, she decided to keep them. I can't remember the other mission. I make it sound like a joke. It is not a joke. It is sad, so sad. It is not her fault; she can't help it.

Neither can she make any useful contribution; when she tries it inevitably slows me down. I hate writing this but it's the only alternative to wimping out and telling the family.

Monday 22 December 2014

Christmas is nearly here – and I've had enough. I am feeling wretched and struggling. This journal is turning into the story of the mental and physical decline of the central focus of my life. It is agonising but I can't bring myself to talk about it, nor to seek help.

My poor darling is completely confused. In spite of me telling her several times a day, she has only the vaguest idea of our schedule over Christmas. Jonathan has to fly a planeload of holiday makers to Sharm-el-Sheik on Christmas Day so he and Tracey are giving us Christmas lunch on 23 December. We are spending Christmas Day on our own to save Jeanne too much socialising, and we are going to Sarah on Boxing Day.

Saturday 27 December 2014

What a relief, we are on the other side of Christmas. The lunch on 23 December was lovely but turned sour for me. After only a couple of glasses of wine, I suddenly began to feel and behave as though I was very drunk. Jeanne was very cross with me. Next day I discovered that I had taken a double dose of my diabetes meds. I wasn't drunk – I was hypoglycaemic.

This demonstrated where my head was at the time and the probable cause was all the things that were going through it. I always carry a spare set of meds wherever I go. It was clear that I took those as well as the scheduled dose because both boxes were empty the next day.

We had decided to lunch on our own on Christmas Day to save Jeanne too much socialising. Just as well! Whilst I was serving up the meal, she went into sphinx mode for ten minutes. When she emerged, she left most of her lunch on the plate and had little to say for the rest of the day, apart from criticizing my cooking.

> *NOTE: I can't emphasise too many times that it is not the patient's fault when you are faced with this sort of behaviour. It is not them talking – it is the illness. Dealing with it by remaining placid was one of the most stressful things I have done. Because the patient still looks like the same person it is so easy to take issue with them, but please remember that an hour later their short-term memory will have little or no recollection of it.*

Boxing Day was completely different. We went to Sarah and my darling was as bright as a button, almost like her old self and said, when asked, that we'd enjoyed having a quiet Christmas Day on our own.

> *I felt that no one realised how big a shadow was cast by the ups and downs of her evolving condition, but it seemed pointless to keep banging on about it.*

Wednesday 7 January 2015

Eleven days since my last entry. That shows just how busy my days are. If a vacant few minutes arise, I rarely have enough energy to do any other than fall asleep in my chair. Today we had the phlebotomist again for the next Thyroid Function Test. This was absolutely no problem. What Jeanne is dreading is the follow-up visit to the GP, but not because the TFT result is worrying her: she is afraid he will ask her more of 'those questions' – the MMSE.

> *To put her mind at rest I reminded her about the Memory Gateway. It seemed feasible that if we asked him to refer us for the full assessment programme he*

wouldn't waste time on yet another MMSE. But she
remained terrified – rightly as it turned out.

Monday 12 January 2015

The results of the TFT are satisfactory and the thyroxine dose has been prescribed for the foreseeable future. But I was quite wrong about asking the GP for a referral to the Memory Gateway. This prompted him to run the full MMSE.

The full test attracts a total of 30 points and the patient's score gives a good idea of the degree of cognitive impairment. Jeanne didn't do too badly: the GP said he would give her about 22 out of 30. Had she known the year was 2015, not '1915' (which she said, more in hope than expectation) she might have squeezed one or two more points. Subsequent research shows that 24 upwards is considered normal, 18 to 23 is a mild cognitive impairment – which seemed about right.

He thinks a referral to the Memory Gateway is probably a good idea but warned us not to expect a very prompt response; other patients had reported a wait of at least three months.

When we got home, she was upset because of the way the doctor had been laughing at her while asking the questions. She hadn't realised that he was smiling at her as a way of trying to put her at her ease. It is worth noting that there may have been a certain amount of significance in that, but I'll come to that later.

Tuesday 13 January 2015

As a final thought yesterday, the doctor asked me if we had done anything about granting a Power of Attorney for Jeanne to our children. I haven't. I must crack on with this as a priority.

This was a good point. I had assumed this was unnecessary because our will is a 'survivor takes all' arrangement. But if I should die first, Jeanne would probably not be of sound mind in the legal sense and, without a Power of Attorney, solicitors would have to intervene, at a sizeable cost in terms of both money and time.

Wednesday 14 January 2015

The correct term is Lasting Power of Attorney, commonly known as LPA. It is Jeanne who has to grant the LPA by signing the forms in front of a reliable witness, after which the form has to be signed by a 'responsible but disinterested person' to attest to her being of sound mind at the time.

I could have done without this additional responsibility but it was crucial to get on with it. Our GP was prepared to attest on behalf of Jeanne – AT THAT TIME. A month later and he might have been less convinced. There was no time to lose! Advice on granting the LPA is given in Further Information at the end of the book.

Sunday 25 January 2015

In the meantime, it will soon be spring and the notion of moving has re-surfaced. There is a flat on the market in Swanage which might be worth a look, but I still worry about Jeanne's ability to cope with the change. She moves in and out of 'a dream world' in which she sees all the best bits without seeing the snags. When she comes out of the dream world the exact opposite applies, and there is no way of knowing which world she is in at the time. It is not easy! And, of course, we still have Annie Catt (as she has become known) as part of the equation.

Wednesday 28 January 2015

Jeanne seems to be accepting her problems now but – and it's a big BUT – she cannot be persuaded to share them with anyone else but me. It would make everything so much easier if she could. Most days I find it necessary to help her dress and, indeed, choose what she is going to wear. Oh dear! I often feel like crying for her. It seems so bloody unfair.

> *I was very close to tears when I wrote this; for both of us, for what we have lost and for what I was still desperately trying to hang on to.*

Monday 2 February 2015

We had a big breakthrough yesterday when Sarah came in for a chat. Finally, my lady agreed that it is better to be open about her problems within the family. We persuaded her to ignore the supposed stigma attaching to mental health problems. The conversation caused her lips to quiver a little and the odd tear to drop but, ever since then, she has seemed more relaxed about everything.

Earlier this evening she asked me to speak to Maureen (one of her cousins) to put her in the picture, after which they had a long conversation. Now she wants me to open a call with Doreen (the old school-friend) so that she can talk to her.

Subsequently there was a change of plan. The call to Maureen worked perfectly well but the main point of contacting Doreen was to explain that it would be difficult to have her to stay that summer. We decided an initial letter would be more appropriate, and a whole lot easier, even though it took me a couple of hours to compose!

Tuesday 3 February 2015

Yesterday was the day that the Memory Gateway fiasco came to light. We had heard nothing since 12 January, the day when the GP was alleged to have sent the referral. I rang the Gateway number given on their website. They had no record of the referral. In a subsequent phone call, the Swanage Medical Practice assured me that it had been faxed on 12 January. Back to the Memory Gateway where someone eventually discovered the fax: it was just a blank piece of paper.

This sort of stupidity is unacceptable. It was stupid of Swanage to fax a blank piece of paper, and even more stupid of the Gateway not to check with the fax number that sent a blank piece of paper to see what it was all about. But I couldn't say as much to either organisation: we needed them on our side.

Friday 6 February 2015

A call from the Memory Gateway said that they now had the referral and that an adviser would be allocated to us 'next Monday', 9 February.

Thursday 12 February 2015

The 9 February came and went: we have heard nothing. They have until next Monday by which time my patience will have been exhausted and they will be subjected to a continual bombardment until I get some sense out of them.

I wrote that before a letter from the Memory Gateway arrived the same day. An adviser had been appointed and they will be in touch to arrange a home visit. How long that would take remained to be seen.

Saturday 14 February 2015

Last night we took Sarah and Ems to see the ballet 'Romeo & Juliet', in Poole. Jeanne managed very well: the good thing about ballet is that dancing can be enjoyed for itself without any comprehension of the plot, which would depend on her short-term memory.

We used to enjoy plays in the theatre, but her ability to follow a story line in TV dramas had made this a thing of the past.

Monday 16 February 2015

Nothing so far from the memory adviser but today is Jeanne's eightieth birthday and I don't want to spoil it by having a set-to with those people. Fortunately, she has forgotten all about that stuff: she can just sit back and enjoy her day.

She had flowers and presents from me and all the family, plus visits from Jon and Tracey and Sarah and Paul. Lizzie couldn't make it from Daventry that weekend but, because it was my birthday the following Saturday, she was coming for a mega birthday bash at the Black Swan with as many of the family that could make it.

Tuesday 17 February 2015

Today is recovery day! Not from an excess of booze but there are flowers everywhere and I have to tidy them up. Until quite recently, Jeanne would have dealt with this; her organisational skills now are such that she has no idea where to start. My first thoughts involve the green recycling bin outside, but I'd better see if I can add flower arranging to my skill-set. They actually look quite good. The bigger problem is sending 'thank you' texts on behalf of someone who no longer can do it for herself. I wondered about her sending old-fashioned 'thank you' cards, but her writing would give the game away.

Thursday 19 February 2015

It is no more than a few weeks ago that Jeanne could still work the washing machine; now, even that skill has left her. I have been ironing my shirts to save her the trouble for quite some time, but now the whole laundry job is down to me. There are a couple of loads to plough through, and while the washing is in the machine I am cleaning the kitchen.

> *I told anybody that called in that we were doing early spring cleaning. Actually, it had more to do with the projected move and having to open up the place to estate agents and potential purchasers – if there were going to be any.*

Friday 20 February 2015

Ironing today: it all needs to be out of the way by tomorrow – party day – or, even better, by this afternoon when Sarah is coming to do her Mum's hair.

Saturday 21 February 2015

My birthday! It is now lunchtime at home, for just the two of us, having had coffee and cakes at Sarah's at eleven o'clock with as many of the family that could make it. Now for a restful afternoon before I start to get my lady ready for our joint eightieth birthday party at 'The Black Swan'.

Sunday 22 February 2015

That was a great success. Jeanne didn't have second thoughts about what we'd agreed she was going to wear and, quite amazingly, she was able to walk from the house to the pub. The distance is comfortably within my range but she hasn't walked that far in ages. Again, I begin to feel we have turned a corner.

As far as I can remember the whole family got to the party and Jeanne was, quite simply, the Jeanne we all knew and loved. It was a wonderful evening. The team had clubbed together to buy us an iPad for our joint present which the following day, and unbeknown to any of them, was instrumental in totally destroying my earlier buoyancy. I tried to explain what the iPad was for and how to use it. After trying for an hour, she still hadn't mastered how to turn it on.

Monday 23 February 2015

The Annie Catt problem ended today. Through one of her clients, Sarah had got to hear of a lady who had recently lost a pet and was looking for a replacement. The two ladies came to see us this afternoon and 'Jenny' just loved Annie from the minute she set eyes on her and wanted to take her home with her. Sarah and Ems did the next best thing: they packed up all Annie's bits and pieces plus her store cupboard of food and delivered the whole package to Annie's new home later today. Job done – and, quite unexpectedly, Jeanne was very upset and cried.

Tuesday 24 February 2015

The first morning without Annie. I miss her little face – but not all the extra work that she caused me. But at least she can be removed from the accommodation equation now. I shall be speaking to our estate agents in the near future.

We subsequently heard that Annie was settled in her new home and she and her new owner were very happy with each other.

Still no news from the Memory Gateway. I rang them late afternoon today and spoke to one of the staff who was a bit vague. After a certain amount of kerfuffle, she was able to give me the name of the adviser appointed to our case, and said she would e-mail a reminder straight away. A fat lot of good that that is likely to be!

Wednesday 25 February 2015

I take it all back! The lady adviser was on the phone to me at the crack of dawn and has arranged to visit us at 11.30 on 3 March – this year! Wow!

Thursday 26 February 2015

Jeanne is now in panic mode. I am fearful for her and how she will be, not so much for the actual interview but the time leading up to it. The truth is that she is deteriorating fairly rapidly. It is so tragic and I feel helpless.

NOTE: How could I write that in my diary and still not actively engage the help of my family? I was wearing myself out and, even more importantly, I was depriving Jeanne of an extra line of support in the mistaken belief that 'I had to be strong'.

CHAPTER SIX

Tuesday 3 March 2015

Jeanne was very apprehensive about the visit of the Memory Adviser. I expected the adviser to be helpful and reassuring. For the most part I was right, but even she couldn't resist starting with the dreaded MMSE questions. From there, her line of enquiry was all about how we were managing our everyday lives. She was also an Occupational Therapist and trained to assess whether our home could be made safer by adding grab rails at danger points. Her report would go to the Memory Assessment Officer who would visit us next.

NOTE: A copy of her report reached us many weeks later, by which time it was irrelevant. The content seemed trivial, much of what we told her was misunderstood and it was littered with stupid mistakes. Jeanne's name was spelled correctly only once: after that it was consistently given as Jean. My name alternated between Brian and Barry throughout the report. I doubt if it had been read by anyone.

We are going to look at a McArthy & Stone apartment tomorrow. I have no idea if Jeanne will be able to cope with such a move, but it has to be considered if only because of the presence of an onsite manager and the Careline support system.

McArthy & Stone specialize in owner-occupied flats for the older generation with a minimum age of 55 years. This particular development was built about 18 years ago on the site where Swanage's Corrie Hotel once stood.

Wednesday 4 March 2015

Sarah, and Jonathan and Tracey came with us to view the apartment. I had an open mind, but was expecting it to be a bit like a care home. The agent had warned me it was not everyone's cup of tea.

Far from being like a care home, the whole complex feels like a really nice hotel. The view from the apartment is spectacular, which accounts for the asking price which is equally spectacular. The corridors are carpeted and heated. The onsite manager, whom we met, is charming and there are Careline pull-cords in every room. We all agreed that it would do us rather well. Part of the difficulty is trying to evaluate Jeanne's opinion. Her mind is not sufficiently well-organised to think it through. I shall take her back for another look, but on our own next time.

Thursday 5 March 2015

Today was my over-75 check-up with the GP. It was mainly about my diabetes and dietary changes that might reduce some of the spikes in my blood sugars. I agreed to give it a try, but the stress of being a full-time carer in a worsening situation is the most likely cause.

We went on to talk a little about Jeanne's condition. I think he was trying to prepare me for a firm diagnosis of Alzheimer's disease. I am not convinced that this is an inevitable outcome.

Saturday 7 March 2015

We took another look at the McArthy & Stone apartment this afternoon, just the two of us this time, plus the estate agent. I think the asking price is fixed more in hope than expectation, but I would be prepared to make a sensible offer. First, I must make a scale drawing to make sure we will fit into what is a smaller space.

This sort of thing is within my professional skill set and took only an hour or two to accomplish. I was satisfied that it would work for us.

Tuesday 10 March 2105

We took a final look at the apartment late afternoon because we have seen it only in the morning up until now, and the windows all face east. We also had Paul with us to give his down-to-earth opinion, and without anyone from the estate agency to inhibit us. We have decided to go ahead with my proposed offer, so I shall speak to the agents tomorrow.

Wednesday 11 March 2105

Good news! The agents have revised the asking price for our house upwards so my offer reflects that, and is nearer to the sellers' asking price than I had envisaged. The ball is now in the agents' court. I can forget about it for a few days. How will it affect Jeanne? We had a long talk about it yesterday but she finds difficulty in remembering all the 'ifs' 'buts' and 'maybes' of our previous experience in the property market.

With regard to the offer, my position was quite simple. The difference between our selling price and the apartment buying price had to cover all costs. I didn't want the move to cost any of our savings.

Wednesday 18 March 2015

The agents have been in to take photos and measurements prior to advertising our house and printing the leaflets.

Tuesday 24 March 2105

We've started! The agents brought the first viewers to look at the house yesterday. They liked it immediately and asked to come back for a second look later the same day. Today they made an offer which is a bit on the low side so the agents have suggested a more appropriate figure to them, after which they talked to the agents selling the apartment to see how much room we have for negotiation.

Tuesday 1 April 2015

The house business is now out of my control so Jeanne and I have slipped back into our normal routine. She bought a puzzle book a few days ago, probably to prove to herself that she could still do puzzles. She gave up after about 15 minutes. Recently she suggested a game of Scrabble. Because it was of the past, I thought she would be OK. No luck there either.

Her recall of past events is still 100%; 'how to do' knowledge, even from her past, is slipping away. I have no idea what to do for the best – and I am shattered.

Watching this lovely woman disintegrate is pitiful, and it appears that nothing can be done to reverse the process.

I have to keep my spirits up, for her sake, for everybody's sake – while the help we need is so pathetically slow in reaching us.

Friday 3 April 2015

I have been up since 05.45. Our prospective buyers are coming back for a third look at the house at 11.00 today and my lady didn't feel up to seeing them. The agents had no one available, so Sarah is standing in for us. It means that we need to be out of the house by 10.30 and it takes that long to get Jeanne dressed. I can't leave her to do it herself, because she no longer knows where to start.

It was this same morning that she decided there was something wrong with her prescribed remedy for indigestion. She wouldn't take the first pill because it was stuck in the container and the second one she just spat out. On reflection, the truth is that sometimes she was beginning to inhabit a private world that made perfect sense to her, but none whatsoever to me.

It was my job to keep her happily on an even keel, without revealing my inner struggle, without losing my patience and at no time laughing at her problems.

What a good job Sarah did see the intending buyers: they stayed for an hour and twenty minutes. This would have exceeded Jeanne's attention span, and would have put mine under threat. But they were very nice and left presents for us of a miniature rose and box of chocolates.

Saturday 4 April 2015

That's it! The deal has been done. Our viewers have become our buyers with a very respectable offer and an assurance that they are in no hurry to complete: they are buying it for their retirement and are going to let it out in the meantime. Even better, the executors for the apartment have agreed to my offer on the basis that we have a firm offer that is not dependent on a chain behind us. Everything is pointing in the right direction; I think it was meant to happen. But Jeanne's illness remains the defining cloud that dampens my enthusiasm. Managing the move alongside my caring role is going to be a challenge.

But I was determined to present a relaxed attitude. If you ask me now, it would be hard to explain why. The probable answer is bloody-mindedness!

I was also sorting out the three sets of forms granting Lasting Power of Attorney as a matter of urgency:

a) the GP couldn't sign them as our 'certificate provider' until they had been signed by the Attorneys, each in the presence of a witness who knew them but who was independent;

b) the GP's signature was on condition he agreed Jeanne was still mentally aware enough to know what she was signing – and there was little doubt her faculties were diminishing quite rapidly;

c) I might need one of the Attorneys to sign on Jeanne's behalf when we get to the conveyancing stage: she is no longer happy signing her own name.

Tuesday 7 April 2015

Jeanne has been unexpectedly more at ease since the deal has been agreed. It may be that she was being stressed by not knowing – or maybe there is no reason at all.

Monday 13 April 2015

I seem to be in a vacuum, waiting for other people. We've had no report yet from the Memory Adviser, nor when the Memory Assessment Nurse is coming. The LPA papers are with the GP and I am waiting to hear that they are ready for collection. We have received the Memorandum of Sale from the estate agents, so all that is in the hands of our solicitors.

Wednesday 15 April 2015

The first pile has arrived from the solicitors, the most daunting of which is the Property Information Form on which we have to give details of the contents and fixtures included in the sale. To my surprise, and even greater pleasure, Jeanne has been helping me with it; of course, a lot of it concerns past history.

I should have known from experience that it wouldn't last long: later that evening she went back into her shell. It wasn't quite sphinx mode but she had lost her earlier enthusiasm for helping. On reflection, she may have been tired.

Monday 20 April 2015

Today was very difficult. The stress of our potential move is getting to her; her inability to remember anything I say is getting to me. It does get very wearing when you have a lot to think about – and I do have a lot to think about. Sometimes I feel very forlorn . . .

Tuesday 21 April 2015

Today was much better. I started bringing things out of the loft, mainly old children's games and playthings. We cast judgement on them: 'keep' or 'dump'! She really enjoyed that; definitely a nostalgia trip, which is right up her street. It was mostly 'dump' so the car is full of stuff for the Recycling Centre.

Friday 24 April 2015

Just when everything seemed to be going so well – along comes the bombshell! The estate agents called late this afternoon to say that they had just heard that the executors for the sale of the apartment had accepted an offer from another potential buyer alongside ours. In other words, it is now a 'contract race'.

> *It would have been kinder if the agents had kept this to themselves until after the weekend. It messed up my darling big time: the equilibrium I had managed to establish was shattered in seconds and there was nothing I could do until Monday.*

Monday 27 April 2015

The agents called me to say that they will underwrite any financial losses if we fail to win the contract race. Over the weekend I had made up my mind: the stress of a contract race is more than either of us could stand. The agents, of course, know nothing of Jeanne's problems but they have agreed to ring the executors' solicitors to say that we are out of the race.

Tuesday 28 April 2015

A good decision! We have been gazumped! The new bidders have offered the full asking price, which is more than I am prepared to pay. I am cross because it is unethical, but secretly I am relieved – and amused. If the bidders hadn't been in such a hurry they could have saved themselves a goodish sum of money! Even Jeanne could see the funny side of that.

> *I was relieved on two counts. Firstly, I felt that the asking price was excessive, and even my offer was far more than was justified by the quality of the accommodation, and the amount that needed doing to it. Secondly, since I made the offer there had already been sufficient deterioration in Jeanne's condition that I was unsure whether I could manage both her and the proposed move.*

CHAPTER SEVEN

Thursday 30 April 2015

Yesterday afternoon we looked at another flat in the hands of different agents. It seems worth having a second look today, with Sarah.

> *In spite of Jeanne's worsening condition, I was keen to keep on the trail because our buyers had made a good offer, had a completely flexible timescale and were nice people. I didn't want to let them down.*

Friday 1 May 2015

That viewing went rather well and we were joined by Jonathan as well as Sarah. It seems a better proposition than the one we've just lost. The first-floor accommodation is more spacious and laid out more thoughtfully. It is approached by a dedicated staircase with a chair lift, which Jeanne finds perfectly acceptable. A few things need fixing but the asking price is within budget so not a problem.

We think we shall go for it, but the weekend starts tomorrow and my lady is nicely relaxed so we are giving ourselves a couple of days off.

Sunday 3 May 2015

Some of my worries about moving came creeping back over the weekend. What is wearing is trying to decide what to discuss with Jeanne to cause her the least amount of stress, how to discuss it and to judge the best time to raise the subject.

Knowing how much she was likely to remember was also a bit of a teaser. Although this was our seventh move coming up, the procedures involved in conveyancing were a complete mystery to her.

Thursday 7 May 2015

Our surveyor has given the flat a clean bill of health, apart from a squeaky floor which the estate agents are going to get a local builder to assess.

Saturday 9 May 2015

Earlier today Jeanne was in one of her more lucid moments. She began to wonder if there was a connection between her seemingly random symptoms.

I suggested we make a list and enter the items into Google. This is it.

1. Her writing is lacking its traditional neatness and is noticeably smaller.
   I hadn't been sure she was aware of this, but it was the first thing she mentioned.
2. She is speaking more quietly.
   This was something that was more evident to me than her, particularly in the car.
3. Her posture is deteriorating and she is developing a pronounced stoop.
   We were inclined to attribute this to troublesome knees, one of which had been replaced in 2012.
4. Her balance has become impaired.
   There had been several falls, and near-misses where she had managed to save herself, or I had been able to save her. These may have been due to the same knee trouble.

5. The short-term memory loss.
   *This was her preferred description of the more
   accurate 'mild cognitive impairment'.*

Google took us to:
    'The 10 Most Common Symptoms of Parkinson's
Disease'.
    I almost whooped in triumph! I hadn't thought of
that one. I know precious little about it but people with
Parkinson's seem to live a normal life span.

> *There were some signs and symptoms which Jeanne
> didn't have, the most obvious being the distinctive
> tremor. Apparently about 30% of patients don't
> develop the tremor at onset, and some don't have it
> at all. (She also said she had lost her sense of smell but
> that doesn't seem to be a symptom of Parkinson's.)*

> *Jeanne's reaction to our findings could only
> be described as grumpy. Mine was pure relief.
> Parkinson's seems to be manageable with medication;
> it is not known to cause unacceptable pain and, most
> importantly, is not regarded as terminal.*

> *Within a day or so she came to see things my way.
> She seemed closer to me than she had been for some
> time as she accepted that it was much better to
> suffer from a known illness, that we could deal with
> together, than to suffer with a load of symptoms
> that might mean almost anything.*

Monday 11 May 2015

There was a lot of nostalgia on TV over the weekend: it
was the seventieth anniversary of VE Day. Jeanne enjoyed
it and it kept her from dwelling on her problems.

This morning I arranged a phone appointment with our GP for tomorrow at 3.30pm.

There was a response from the Memory Gateway today: it will be another three weeks before the next visit!

Tuesday 12 May 2015

The GP agreed the symptoms could indicate Parkinson's disease. He has given us an appointment for next Monday. In the meantime, I have been reading a book by a woman with Parkinson's: it makes so much sense as a diagnosis I am almost convinced!

Jeanne is terrified: I don't think that's too strong a word. We've talked a lot about her feelings and, typically, her biggest worry is "What will people think?" There is no shame attaching to the condition. What I want her to think is that Parkinson's is life-changing but NOT life-threatening. But there is some way to go. First, we have to see the GP. My hope is he'll refer us to a specialist.

Wednesday 13 May 2015

Time for lunch out – and some much-needed retail therapy.

After lunch, we hit the shops: F&F in Tesco, two pairs of trousers; George in Asda, at least six pairs of trousers; M&S, a bra and top; Primark, six tops.

This evening we have been trying things on: everything is going back tomorrow – the whole bloody lot! But she enjoyed her day . . .

Thursday 14 May 2015

I collated all the Lasting Power of Attorney forms, checked them, and they are on their way to the Office of the Public Guardian for registration.

Friday 15 May 2015

The carpet layer will fix the squeaky floors at the flat as part of his job. Now that is sorted I have made an offer. The agents say that the vendors would like £5k more. I've suggested we split the difference. The weekend is on us so it will be Monday before we know if we are in a 'go' situation. Never mind, I have washing, ironing and cleaning to pass the time, but first it's off to John Lewis. All of which is actually quite relaxing compared with most of what I do.

We were half way home from John Lewis when I had a call from the vendors' agents to say that my offer to split the difference has been accepted. We're off again and the thing I liked most of all was Jeanne saying: "This is fun!" just like she would have done in what I now think of as 'the old days'.

Monday 18 May 2015

The GP wasn't entirely convinced by my Parkinson's diagnosis, probably because of the absence of the characteristic tremor. But he thought he could detect evidence of what is known as a 'cogwheel motion' in her arms that was sufficient for him to refer us to a geriatric consultant who specialises in movement disorders.

At the time, I struggled with understanding cogwheel motion, which is also known as cogwheel rigidity. I now know that the patient is rarely aware of it; it has no significant effect on their everyday life, but has diagnostic significance. It is best described as alternating resistance and release of movement, when being manipulated by an experienced doctor, usually in the wrists, elbows and ankles.

Friday 22 May 2015

We are still waiting for the Memorandum of Sale. It has been held up by the fact that the executors of the deceased owner of the flat are a firm of solicitors, not the people inheriting. The executors want to do the conveyancing themselves; the vendors wish to use their own solicitors. Meanwhile, we sit drumming our fingers.

Saturday 23 May 2015

A good day today. The Memorandum of Sale arrived. It has no legal standing but shows that everyone is ready to proceed. In the same post, there was a letter from Poole Hospital with Jeanne's appointment to see the consultant about her suspected Parkinson's disease on 10 June and, even better, at Swanage Hospital.

Sunday 24 May 2015

I had a sound sleep last night, the first for a long time. Now I feel exhausted. It has been an effort to keep going and keep my humour in good repair. I need a rest, but I'm not going to get much of one until the move is over.

I read frequently about carers needing respite: I have been caring for two years, almost three, and beginning to wonder when and how it can be achieved. Jeanne is so dependent on me that she is not happy for me to go down town without her – but it takes ages to get her ready. She is just as fastidious about her appearance as ever; but this, of course, is a good thing.

If I do slip out for ten minutes to get a few bits and pieces, she is waiting by the back door for me to come in. What if she should go out into the garden on her own? There are uneven steps and jagged edges of Purbeck stone everywhere. Even worse, she could go wandering about in the road looking for me? I am desperately worried. What should I do? Obviously, I can't lock her in. I feel I should talk to the family, but they have enough to do already without being dragged into my problems.

Monday 25 May 2015

I wrote that last night. I feel much better this morning and, in some ways, wish I hadn't written it; but probably it needs to be known that, as much as I like to think otherwise, I am NOT indomitable!

Sarah is coming for coffee at 11.00; Jeanne wanted us to be up soon after six "because there isn't much time". Alas this is true. She said to me yesterday that she goes into the bathroom to wash – and doesn't know what to do. It is so sad.

Sunday 31 May 2015

Our solicitors tell me that the freeholders of the flat are going into liquidation. What that means to us is not at all clear – so why bother to tell me? I have enough problems already. I am carrying on as though there is no significance.

> NOTE: Trivial issues like this seemed to crop up all the time. Learning how to deal with them calmly is imperative if you are to keep your patient out of 'stress land', and it's essential that you do.

Wednesday 3 June 2015

Jeanne started the day badly. She spent most of the night worrying about her symptoms: she believes they are getting worse. What can I do to reassure her – when I think she is right?

My medical knowledge depends on the internet plus the few Kindle books I have acquired. I need a support system.

How do I get one? It is so very frustrating. I had high hopes of the Memory Gateway – but they are not cutting it.

It will be a relief to see the consultant next week.

Sunday 7 June 2015

Lizzie came down to stay with Sarah on Friday for a weekend with the team. We ate with them on Friday and Saturday evenings. Everything seemed completely normal. Am I exaggerating the difficulties?

Monday 8 June 2015

Our buyers' surveyor came today. He was with us for two-and-a-half hours and did a full survey rather than just a value-for-money job. Very relieved when he was kind enough to say on leaving that he had nothing adverse to report.

Wednesday 10 June 2015

Today we saw the consultant to get an expert opinion on Jeanne's symptoms.

The consultant has a clinic in our local hospital so we were spared the need to go to Poole Hospital where it's extremely difficult to park and even more difficult to find the venue in a network of corridors that all look the same.

The consultant was very thorough, treated Jeanne gently and with respect. He concluded that she probably has Parkinson's disease. He will report his diagnosis to our GP and ask him to issue us with a prescription for a drug called Madopar, to treat her physical symptoms.

For administrative reasons, the GP had to write the actual prescription. This seems to be in line with usual NHS practice.

There are drugs to treat the mental symptoms but these must be prescribed by a psychiatrist. The first consultant will be passing the case over to an appropriate consultant to oversee that part of Jeanne's treatment.

The Parkinson's consultant apologised for this necessity. In his opinion, because Jeanne's mental difficulties were part of the overall condition, it should have been within his remit to prescribe for them. Clearly, he felt strongly about this. I think I understand why. It was inevitable that handover would add several days, possibly weeks, before she would be treated for what was her most significant disability.

The best news is that we will have access to the Parkinson's support network, manned by four nurse practitioners. We need a referral from our GP: from then on, we will be only a phone call away from help.

Just before we left, the consultant said something about Lewy Bodies that I didn't quite hear. I should have queried it but Jeanne was getting restless and showing signs of wanting to leave.

I now know a great deal more about why the Parkinson's diagnosis was 'probable' and why Lewy Bodies were mentioned. Lewy Bodies are abnormal aggregates of protein that develop inside the brain and can be identified only under a microscope post-mortem. They are always present in Parkinson's disease but also occur in other less well-known

diseases in which case the symptoms are known as Parkinsonism, which is a syndrome characterised by a combination of any of the movement disorders seen in Parkinson's disease, but doesn't include cognitive impairment.
There will be more about this later.

I left feeling happy even though Jeanne has been diagnosed with a disease for which there is still no cure. The point is that it is not life-threatening within the accepted understanding of the term – and it is not Alzheimer's disease from which there appears to be no future that doesn't include total cognitive impairment.

CHAPTER EIGHT

Tuesday 16 June 2015

This morning Sarah arranged some respite for me. She took Jeanne for coffee to our local garden centre while I went to the beach to draw the fishing boats – and associated paraphernalia. It was good to concentrate on something different.

Jeanne was interested in my drawings: her comments were as probing as ever – and valid. This convinces me that she is not on the Alzheimer's trail.

Afterwards I asked Sarah how her Mum had been. She felt it wasn't a huge success, mainly because Jeanne had been worrying about me most of the time, and wondering why I hadn't gone with them.

NOTE: She asked Sarah why I needed time on my own. There was more behind this question than I realised at the time.

Wednesday 17 June 2015

It is now a week since we saw the consultant and still nothing from our GP. I rang the practice two days ago: they are still waiting to hear from the consultant. Today I was more persistent. The switchboard put me through to the medical secretaries. They put me through to the medical secretaries at Swanage Hospital who confirmed that they had typed everything the day after our appointment and sent it to Poole Hospital for the consultant's signature. So far it hasn't come back, but the secretaries have faxed an unsigned copy to our GP, so that he can get things moving.

Thursday 18 June 2015

The draft contract arrived from our solicitors this morning. No time to look at it today: we have to take the car to Poole for its annual service.

Monday 22 June 2015

I can't believe it! I've read the contract. It shows that the stairlift, that is essential to our purchase, was installed by the previous owner without permission. The freeholders agreed to it remaining only on condition that when that owner left the flat the stairlift was removed and the staircase made good. I've spoken to our solicitor. I really haven't time to see if it's possible to negotiate, and bearing in mind the rumour that the freeholders are going into liquidation, I've pulled the plug on this deal. Start again – again!

> *It was good that our buyers were prepared to wait for as long as it takes, but starting again when there was so much else to worry about was maddening. I might easily have given up on the whole project, but there were three considerations.*
>
> a) *Our buyers so loved our house that they were prepared to wait indefinitely.*
> b) *The stairs and the garden were such a threat to Jeanne's safety that it would have been irresponsible to give up.*
> c) *Jeanne liked looking at property. It kept her mind on things other than her ailments and looking at property was the sort of cloud-cuckoo land she was comfortable with, compared with the nitty-gritty business of actually buying it, which was no longer in her territory.*

Tuesday 23 June 2015

Jeanne's new medication, Madopar, for the movement disorders associated with Parkinson's disease, has arrived – almost two weeks since we saw the consultant.

Tuesday 30 June 2015

Jeanne is on three doses of Madopar a day which, little by little, seem to be improving how she feels.

Yesterday, we saw a much better apartment in the McArthy & Stone development. The layout is more suitable, and it is in excellent condition. It has no sea view but is £80,000 less than the previous one. Jeanne was having one of her really good days and loved it. I rang the agents as soon as we were home and offered the full asking price. The offer was accepted within the hour. The agents have marked it 'SOLD – subject to contract', and taken the property off the market.

Unfortunately, as I've said before, Jeanne had forgotten how tortuous conveyancing can be and seemed to think we would be moving in a couple of weeks.

Sunday 5 July 2015

Over the last day or two, I fell to a vicious bug (probably aggravated by stress).

This morning Jeanne brought me a cup of tea in bed. I was thrilled. Before Madopar, her movement disorders would have made this quite impossible.

Everything to do with the flat purchase seems to be going well. I'm certain this one is going to happen, and we shall be in by the autumn.

Tuesday 7 July 2015

Jeanne has started to show signs of what can be best described as paranoia. She seems to think that we are being secretly observed: that 'they' are watching everything we do. These thoughts seem more intense at night. Last night, I had a thought of my own: has this started since the introduction of Madopar?

> *I lay awake for ages. I became certain that Madopar was the problem. I checked the literature supplied with the drug: mental disturbances were given as unwanted side-effects – including paranoia. Should I stop it immediately, even though it was helping her movement difficulties – or talk to the GP first? Probably the latter.*

But today we have the Memory Assessor coming; better deal with him first.

He was a nice man, and arrived on time. His assessment was based on three sets of questions, with scores to establish the extent of Jeanne's dementia. She came through it very well, but it was obvious that her scores were not very high.

> *In due course, we received his written report. It was much more professional and clinical in style than that of the Advisor. As I had predicted, her scores were not very encouraging.*

Later the same day

As soon as the Assessor had gone, I tried to talk to a doctor at our medical practice, without success. A medical secretary said to call again the next day if I was still worried. I tried to ring the Parkinson's nurses: there was no reply.

So much for the 'help is only a phone call away'. I am beginning to lose my sense of humour.

Wednesday 8 July 2015

Last night the paranoia was much the same. This morning I called the practice and the first available doctor rang me back. I expounded my Madopar theory. She suggested that we reduce the Madopar from three times a day to twice. She said that she would write to the Parkinson's consultant and to the associated psychiatrist to put them in the picture.

Thursday 9 July 2015

Thank goodness! The reduction of the Madopar dose seems to have done the trick. Today Jeanne appears to be much more relaxed

Saturday 11 July 2015

Today the paranoia became worse. It took a large step in the worst possible direction – it was focused on me.

Overnight she was very frightened. She kept asking: "Why are you doing this to me?" At first, I thought she had awakened from a bad dream, but the situation continued until daybreak.

Later that morning

I told her that it was OK, that I was Brian and she was safe.

She said I wasn't Brian. This shook me to the core.

She said that I looked like Brian, but the voice was wrong; it was a 'funny' voice – like Mickey Mouse. She thought I was an imposter. She thought the imposter had been sent do her harm.

Then she started to warn me, the imposter, that if the real Brian comes back and finds 'you' here he will get very nasty. I believe it was the only strategy she could think of that might get rid of the imposter.

Early afternoon

It is a desperate time. I am scared for her; I am terrified for me. The agony of responsibility is stacking up on my shoulders, remorselessly. There seems no end to it. I am her carer, but she no longer trusts me. What do I do?

All I can do is try to be as normal as possible and carry on with the usual routines. Somehow, we struggled through the morning; how I can't remember.

I have made a unilateral decision to stop the Madopar completely. Gradually the paranoia seems to be subsiding. I may have won the battle.

Mid-evening

It has started all over again. I have no idea what to do. I can't go through another night like this. I need help.

I called Sarah. She and Paul were both available and arrived within minutes. Their very presence brought a sense of calm and a degree of order to the night ahead of us. They called for a paramedic who was sympathetic but unable to help. His advice was to call 111 and ask for a doctor. Sarah decided to stay for the night which was hugely reassuring. We decided to delay 111 until the morning.

Sunday 12 July 2015

It's our fifty-seventh wedding anniversary. I bought a card, from us to us, which pleased her; and some flowers, of course. There is nothing else to celebrate.

At about five am, I had to wake Sarah. Jeanne had become so paranoid about me that she was holding her hands together as if in prayer, and calling out for her mother, for help. Her mother passed away thirty years ago.

Sarah did as the paramedic suggested. She called 111, explained the situation and asked for a doctor.

NOTE: This was excellent advice and well worth bearing in mind in this sort of situation.

An emergency doctor arrived mid-morning. He immediately suspected the cause to be a urinary tract infection (UTI). A specimen was produced which he dipped: the result confirmed his suspicions. He was able to dispense an antibiotic from his bag (two per day for three days), and said we should speak to our GP tomorrow.

This was a new one on me: I had no idea that a UTI could lead to mental disturbances.

As soon as possible I was on the internet: sure enough, there it was. AgingCare.com confirmed that in elderly people the most likely consequences of a UTI are behavioural, such as becoming confused – or PARANOID! Further research confirmed that the side effects of taking Madopar can also lead to paranoia.

A double whammy – great!

Early evening

The paranoia went almost immediately. Sarah and Paul were able to go home soon after. My beloved Jeanne seems to have forgotten the paranoid delusions. We have settled back into our normal routine. Relief!

Monday 13 July 2015

I slept for eight hours. Absolute heaven! At about eleven am today I was able to speak to our GP, as suggested by the emergency doctor. I had assumed that the antibiotics we had been given were just to tide us over until the practice and the pharmacy were open. Not so: two a day for three days is the usual treatment.

I told the GP that I had stopped giving her Madopar on the basis of my reading on the internet. He agreed we leave it out for a few days, and to re-introduce two a day on Friday. If it seems OK, resume three a day after the weekend.

He also said he would like a urine specimen to go to Poole Hospital for analysis to make certain of the source of the UTI.

Things were going fine until early evening. Jonathan was visiting when Jeanne lost her balance on the stairs and fell. Luckily it was from no great height. She was OK. The little table at the foot of the stairs broke her fall – then disintegrated. The fall may have been caused by stopping the Madopar. There were no further incidents. Jonathan was able to leave us – with the remains of the little table to reassemble.

Wednesday 15 July 2015

We've had a couple of delusion-free days. But her delusions have been replaced by worries, most of which are understandable. Top of the list is constipation, for which I have bought a number of different remedies which seem to work, but they don't stop her worrying about it. It is all very wearing.

The good news is that the first bundle from our solicitor arrived today. Jonathan sat with Jeanne to give me time to read through everything. I returned to them with a smile on my face. There is nothing to stop the transaction going through.

Thursday 16 July 2015

Last night, about 2am, she had another fall, this time in the bathroom. She didn't come to any harm which is more than can be said of my back after lifting her up.

My job as carer is getting harder.

I have to start considering getting outside help – but the idea won't go down very well with Jeanne, I'm sure.

After more consideration, I decided to continue on my own, for as long as possible, certainly until after we had moved. I reasoned that the conveyancing should take only a few weeks and that, in a different environment and not one we have built together over a number of years, it should be easier for her to come to terms with a daily visit, or two, from a professional career. Slightly obscure reasoning, but I do know how Jeanne's mind works, or used to work. Perhaps, against my usual instincts, I'm just exercising the soft option – by delaying the hard option.

Friday 17 July 2015

She was not well again this morning. Not paranoid but I felt that the UTI was still causing her trouble. I managed to procure a specimen from her, but too late to send it to Poole Hospital. Our GP kindly saw me for long enough to dip it and agree there was some infection still present. Another course of antibiotics – and we are re-starting Madopar today as well. Here goes . . .

Saturday 18 July 2015

This morning (3am) there seemed to be a huge improvement, and this was maintained throughout the day.

Sunday 19 July 2015

The day started off well enough after a reasonably good night. The constipation problem wasn't a problem at all – but the worry that it might be a problem was a problem in itself.

> *This sounds quite barmy I know, but I include it because it shows how normal everyday things have taken a step away from reality, and how these worries are lurking in the background for most of my day.*

Monday 20 July 2015

Yesterday evening, producing a urine specimen for sending to the hospital today became a problem. It was eventually resolved at 01.45.

> *NOTE: This was indicative of another of Jeanne's troubles: she had become dehydrated. Dehydration in elderly people is another condition that – guess what? You're right! It can cause paranoid delusions! It turns out to be a triple whammy.*
>
> *Dehydration would have aggravated the constipation as well. I tried to encourage her to drink more water, but she had no great enthusiasm for it. Never has.*

The paranoid delusions returned soon after the specimen was produced. I had to call Sarah at the crack of dawn to help me get Jeanne back on what passes as an even keel. Jonathan took the urine specimen to the Path Lab at Poole Hospital for analysis.

> *Our GP responded to a request for a phone call mid-morning and visited us at 1.00pm. He agreed to stop the Madopar and to wait until he had the results from the urine sample before re-starting it.*

The delusions came and went. As the day progressed they became less paranoid and were replaced by hallucinations. She thought she could hear me talking to people in the kitchen which worried her. She wondered who had let a dog into the house. Then she could hear children in the background. This put her mind at rest.

> NOTE: *As a result of talking to our grandson, Luke, the doctor, I know now that there are precise definitions of hallucinations and delusions; previously I have assumed that the two words are interchangeable. They are not.*
>
> *Hallucinations are where someone sees, hears, smells, tastes or feels things that don't exist outside of their own mind.*
>
> *Delusions are where someone has an unshakeable belief in something that is untrue.*
>
> *Both terms come under the general heading of Psychosis. Psychosis also includes confused and disturbed thoughts, lack of insight and lack of self-awareness.*

Tuesday 21 July 2015

A much better start to the day. Tracey came early with our medications: she had collected them from the pharmacy. I had washing and cleaning to do so she sat with Jeanne for a while. As far as I could judge she was absolutely normal with Tracey. What a relief!

After lunch, I involved Jeanne with some things relating to our forthcoming move. The main thing was to go through her 'giant' handbag. It has survived some sixty years since she was a student nurse. It was packed with what we will call memorabilia. Rubbish would have been a better word. It was treated as such.

But she loved going back to the time her memory recalls with stunning accuracy. Suddenly we were the couple we always were. I loved that.

Wednesday 22 July 2015

At our GP practice, if a sample goes off for analysis and the patient hears nothing, it can be assumed that everything is normal. I understand the practice doesn't want to be bombarded with calls, but the result of the UTI test should determine where we go from here. I had to call the practice.

The sample showed that Jeanne was now free from infection. So, what now? I have asked for a priority call from our GP: the earliest I can get is Friday.

Friday 24 July 2015

The call came at half-past nine. The GP said that the test shows Jeanne to be clear of the UTI, but dehydrated. Nothing needs to be done, other than to persuade her to drink more water – if possible.

But she is not well. She is still suffering from delusions; she still has symptoms of Parkinson's disease – and she can do precious little for herself. Had the GP heard anything from the geriatric consultant who wanted her to go on Madopar? No.

I forget how the priority call ended but at this point Jonathan was available and he had had enough. He spoke to the consultant's secretary. Soon after, a Parkinson's nurse rang me to say that the consultant would pay us a home visit – on Monday. Consultant? Home visit? That is what we call a result!

Monday 27 July 2015

Up at the crack of dawn to prepare for the visit. Lizzie arrived yesterday. She and Sarah came in for coffee and to talk about the impending visit, and what we wanted to achieve. We waited; we waited some more. The phone call came mid-afternoon: the consultant's car has broken down – he won't be able to visit today.

Instead, he has fitted us into his clinic at Poole Hospital tomorrow at 3.45pm.

This was just a bit too much for my battle-weary sense of humour. Surely a consultant is important enough to have access to a reliable car.

Never mind, Jeanne quite likes hospitals; as an ex-nurse, she understands them and their staff. Although a year or two ago, when her critical senses were still in good order, she often wished that nurses still dressed like nurses, then she could be sure of who she was talking to: was it a Sister, a Staff Nurse – or a cleaner?

Tuesday 28 July 2015

I had a few spare minutes this morning, so spoke to our solicitor. Is all in order with the proposed move? A reassuring 'Yes'. Thank goodness. After two abortive attempts, Jeanne is convinced that this one will fall through as well.

Lizzie and Sarah came with us to the hospital and helped us find our way to the Yellow Clinic. Just as well. I can never find my way around most hospitals, but Poole is especially tricky.

The consultant was on time. He was happy with Jeanne's physical condition but decided that she should have no more Madopar until he sees her on 16 September. Almost immediately she started to feel faint and giddy. A quick check showed her blood pressure to be too low.

He advised us to drop amlodipine, atenolol and bendrofluomethiazide from her medication. She had been taking these for some years to treat high blood pressure.

He has sent a referral to a psychiatrist to deal with her mental problems. There seems to be enough people on her case, but I feel vague about the organisation. Our experience so far has left us feeling that it's all a bit random.

Thursday 30 July 2015

I've just had two days tidying up loose ends, the dangling of which can easily be overlooked against Jeanne's deterioration.

I have instructed our surveyor to run his eye over the apartment. I've paid a few bills. The paperwork has been tidied up; I still know where everything is.

I've ordered some clothes for Jeanne from a mail order company. It's the easiest way: she no longer wants to go to the shops.

Jeanne still really enjoys going out in the car; not to anywhere in particular, just tootling along the lanes of Purbeck. That was our afternoon, ending up with an ice cream on the view point along the Studland Road.

Saturday 1 August 2015

Yesterday, following a referral from the geriatric consultant, we had the first phone call from a nurse practitioner at the Community Mental Health Team (CMHT).

He, the nurse practitioner, will be running Jeanne's case initially.

He has been in touch with the Memory Advisory Service.

We can expect an appointment with the psychiatrist in the near future.

At last, things are beginning to come together.

Monday 3 August 2015

The weekend was not as good as I had hoped. All the family are in Swanage, as they usually are at this time of year. We have invitations to meals at the various houses, but Jeanne is becoming severely depressed. She has been reluctant to accept any invitations, but we are managing to put in appearances as required, and for as long as seems reasonable.

Each morning she wakes up in tears. This is torture – almost more than I can bear. We cannot go on like this. How do I get the NHS to take Jeanne's case seriously? The stiff upper lip approach is achieving nothing.

By this time, each day was so hectic that there were no opportunities to make entries in my notebook. My diary shows that I talked to our medical practice about her worsening depression. They had nothing, except the 'Sit and Wait' clinic.

CHAPTER NINE

Tuesday 4 August 2015

A dreadful night. Jeanne was sleepless for most of it. I was sleepless for all of it. She was switching between bouts of paranoid delusion and troughs of depression. I managed to get her through until daybreak, but had to call Sarah and Paul soon after 7.00am.

They came quickly and helped me settle her down but, being a work day, they had to be about their businesses. Jeanne's torment of alternating delusion and depression ended when she dropped off to sleep. Mine continued while I tried to concentrate on our move.

When she woke up she remained dozy but, mercifully, much more relaxed.

Subsequent notes from the CMHT show that she had started taking Quetiapine at about this time. This must have been prescribed the previous day by one of our GP team. It could have accounted for the worsening of her condition; it might have been even worse without the drug. Who knows?

Almost every situation is aggravated by this lack of information. How are carers meant to find out about these things?

Wednesday 5 August 2015

NIGHTMARE!!!

We must have had a phone call from the CMHT because of the next entry. There is no reference to

it in my diary but that isn't surprising given the
pressure I was under.

Thursday 6 August 2015

Mid-morning, we had a home visit from a locum psychiatrist
from the CMHT. Sarah joined us for the visit. He was a
personable doctor who took careful notes of what we had
to say. He recommended: a) that Jeanne should have a
CT scan, b) that she should continue with the low dose of
Quetiapine each night.

As a precaution against the Quetiapine aggravating
her paranoid delusions, he gave me a prescription for
Lorazepam to help calm any excessive agitation.

When he passed the prescription to me, Jeanne said,
knowingly:

"That's it, now you've got what you want, haven't
you?"

"What do you mean?" I asked.

"You've got the piece of paper you need to put me
away!"

This was addressed to me, Brian, her husband of fifty-
seven years; not the imposter. Paranoia is blasting away at
me on a daily basis. All I can do is duck and weave. There
is the occasional lull in the onslaught, but it keeps coming
back – usually when it is least expected and when I am
unprepared for it.

How can she possibly believe such a thing? Can she not
remember all the happiness of our life together? Does she
not realise how much I care about her and how much I am
doing to keep her with me, so that I can look after her?

After the doctor had gone, I tried to reassure her
that I had no intention of 'putting her away'; very
much the opposite. I told her how much I loved her,

that all I wanted to do was to keep her at home and to help her enjoy life.

I don't think she believed a word of it.

Additionally, of course, her reaction showed how little she understood of the doctor's visit or what was going on around her.

Subsequently we received a copy of the locum's report to our GP, covering the key issues we had spoken about and his recommendations for a treatment/care plan which would include a CT scan.

NOTE: I quote from the report:

'In the last few days she has become verbally abusive to her husband and family. She has persecutory beliefs, accusing them of plotting against her. She has also been very restless, talking nonsense and not recognising family members.'

Those few lines summarise where we were at the time but, coming from the pen of a professional, they are bare, clinical statements of fact. There is no indication of how awful it was for her; it does not encompass the strained emotions of her family as we struggled from day to day to contain this monster of a disease. We didn't tell him that recently Jeanne had tried to hit out at Lizzie – for taking my side in some imagined difference of opinion. Seconds later she was in tears and apologising.

Friday 7 August 2015

ANOTHER NIGHTMARE!!!

I have been feeling awful. At one point, I wondered if I was ill: cancer perhaps.

I am ashamed to admit that the thought entered my head that being seriously ill would be a welcome relief: it would allow me to lay down the burden I have been carrying for all this time. It is that bad.

Saturday 8 August 2015

Against this background, and unbeknown to me, Jonathan, Lizzie and Sarah had been able to see what I had been denying to myself: that I was exhausted, at a loss to know what to do for the best – and perilously close to breaking down completely.

Lizzie came down to Swanage on the Friday for what, I assumed, was just a social visit, but I realise now that there was more significance.

The girls arrived to see us mid-morning and I asked, more or less straightaway, if they would sit with their Mum while I took a shower. I haven't managed to find time for about three weeks.

Freshly showered, I took the luxury of walking up the road to buy a paper and on the way back had a few peaceful moments in the Parish Church. It was an attempt to ease my desperately troubled soul and clear my battered brain. I think that my absence may have been a pivotal moment. On my return, Jonathan had arrived.

Sarah has a client who has experience of dementia and has offered to assess whether a respite break in a care home for Jeanne might be beneficial for us both.

She called in this morning and talked to Jeanne. Her opinion is that it would be an appropriate move. She knows of a room available in a care home only five minutes away. I don't remember taking any part in the decision making; I don't think I was capable. It was agreed that she should speak to the owners on our behalf.

This is the worst day of my life.

The minute the lady had gone, I burst into unmanly tears. It showed, even to me, how dangerously close I was to the end of my tether. Why did I cry? Because I had fought battle after battle after battle – but I was losing the bloody war!

After lunch, the girls went to look at the accommodation. They thought it was like a nice hotel, and returned with one of the owners. It was agreed that Jeanne should go for a short but unspecified period of time.

I can remember nothing of the conversation that preceded agreement. Jeanne didn't seem to need a great deal of persuasion and I must have decided that keeping a low profile was the most obvious way to show just how reluctant I was to lose her, even though she would be only a few minutes away.

The girls prepared her to go, and Jonathan went to get his car. She was out in the car, having paid me very little attention, when she suddenly remembered:

"I haven't said goodbye to Dad!"

I was thrilled when the message came back and I ran out to the car to be met with a loving kiss – the best thing that has happened to me for ages.

I finally accepted that it was the right thing for her, but I couldn't have made the decision without Jonathan, Lizzie and Sarah. Thanks, all of you.

Sunday 9 August 2015

I wrote in my diary yesterday that it was the worst day in my life. I was asked not to visit today and have been grieving as though I've lost her, which in many ways I have; but that started a long time ago with little, scarcely perceptible, changes. Whoever would have thought it would lead to this?

Monday 10 August 2015

I started the day feeling as though I was quietly dying, dying from guilt, dying from the guilt I always feel when I take the soft option. Surely, I could have found a few more ounces of strength to keep her with me.

Now I have seen her!

She seems so much better. Obviously, she needed more care than I could give her. Sarah and Ems came too, followed shortly by Jonathan and Tracey. Her room is a comfortable size, with an en-suite bathroom, and sufficient chairs for visitors. The staff brought us drinks: it was all very sociable. I am sitting at home now feeling a whole lot happier. The truth is that I can relax for a few hours; the first time for ages. It wasn't the soft option. It was hard for me, but right for my darling Jeanne.

Tuesday 11 August 2015

Today Jonathan and I took Jeanne to Poole Hospital for the CT scan. This went very well and we had lunch in the hospital restaurant afterwards. She said how much she had enjoyed the day and that she had felt 'almost normal'.

Wednesday 12 August 2015

The level of care in the home is excellent but some of the male residents have what is euphemistically known as 'challenging behaviour'. One of them, who has the manner and accent of a middle ranking army officer, tried to come into Jeanne's room today while I was with her. I told him that it wasn't his room and that he couldn't come in. He tried to pull rank on me, and said: "We'll soon see about that!", and attempted to force an entry. He picked the wrong bloke – on the wrong day.

He went off saying that I had broken every bone in his body. All I actually did was applied gentle but firm resistance to his forceful attempt to wrestle me out of the way. I was also calling for help from the staff, but none arrived. The gentleman was no further trouble throughout Jeanne's stay.

Thursday 13 August 2015

After all that, I had a diabetic hypo in the middle of the night which left me a bit ropey this morning. But everything that needs doing has been done.

I was joined in my afternoon visit by Jonathan and Tracey, and Tracey's Mum. It was quite a nice little tea party in which we had a few laughs; it was quite like old times and I came away feeling very positive.

Saturday 15 August 2015

Jonathan and Tracey joined us for the morning visit and then they took us up into the hills for coffee and cakes at a popular tea room and afterwards for a drive around the Purbecks. Jeanne absolutely loved it.

Sunday 16 August 2015

I want Jeanne to feel that she can call me at any time whilst she is in the care home. Today I took her the simple phone I bought her a little while ago. She can call me, or any of our three children, by pressing only two keys. At the time, she couldn't grasp the essentials so, before my morning visit, I spent time writing very simple instructions, in large letters. I hope she will be able to do it herself, but if she can't she needs only to show the instructions to a member of staff and they will be able to do it for her.

I spent time going through it with her this morning, until Sarah joined us for coffee. It seemed that she might be able to manage it at the time but less likely this afternoon. This evening she called me but needed one of the staff to help her.

The main reason she called seemed to be that one of the male residents was making too much noise. It hadn't occurred to her that she could have told that to the member of staff who helped make the call – and cut out the middle man!

In due course, I realised that there was a hidden agenda behind her call: but that comes later in the story.

Wednesday 19 August 2015

It's been a busy day or two. When I visited Jeanne on Monday I had ample evidence of the disturbance caused her by the noisy man. It was sufficient for me to make a formal complaint to the staff. Her stay is costing me a lot of money: I expect them to make her feel safe. I was assured the message would be passed to the management.

It was around this time that Jeanne started to talk of another psychotic episode which was part hallucination and part delusion. When we visited she thought there were other people in the room who were helping us to make a film of her. The purpose of the film never became apparent to us, but paranoia was never far away.

Meanwhile Jonathan and I were beginning to think it was high time we heard from the psychiatrist: the CT scan was a week ago. He managed to run the psychiatrist's PA to earth and discovered that they were still waiting for the radiologist's report on the scan. He rang the CT unit at Poole Hospital. They said that it was likely to be another week before the radiologist's report was released.

I think perhaps we were being a bit impatient; it easy to be critical but we have no idea of the workload that falls on these various consultants, nor of the triage assessment of the urgency of all their various commitments.

Because of the noisy men at the care home, Jonathan and I went to look at another care home in town. It was bigger, and quieter, but in every other respect it was inferior. I think to get ideal accommodation without the 'challenging behaviour' element, we will have go further afield.

By this time, it seemed that our move was going ahead quickly and increasingly certain that I would soon have her home with me. However, very sensibly, Lizzie and Sarah visited several care homes in the Bournemouth area to test the market. They were excellent – but a great deal more expensive!

This afternoon the removal company came to give me a price for the move. I am asking them to do all of the packing as well: I really can't undertake that amongst everything else that needs to be done.

Thursday 20 August 2015

I spoke to our GP earlier today about the care home. His said that the level of care was excellent but he did understand that some of the other residents could be difficult. He agreed that the ideal home is not available locally.

Jeanne phoned me after lunch; whether she did it all herself or was helped was unclear, even to her. The main reason for the call seemed to be an 'upset tummy': once again, hardly a problem for the middle man. I was expecting her to be below par for the afternoon visit. When I got to her she was in good spirits and better in every way. I came away feeling very positive.

Friday 21 August 2015

Our proposed move is beginning to look like a certainty. Today I signed various significant papers and Sarah signed for her Mum using the Lasting Power of Attorney. Our solicitor is hoping to exchange contracts today but has been unable to contact the vendor's solicitors.

> *NOTE: I remain grateful to our GP for alerting us to the need for Power of Attorney. By this time, Jeanne was no longer able to sign her own name; when the Power of Attorney was granted she still could. That had changed in no more than a couple of months; her condition was advancing at a frightening rate.*

Saturday 22 August 2015

Our copy of the letter from the Community Mental Health Team to our GP regarding the visit of the locum doctor on 6 August arrived today. The three-page letter was dictated the day of the visit but not typed until 17 August so it is clear that the support staff of the team have a heavy workload.

> *The letter is an accurate description of the situation as it was then. It was the first time that we had*

seen a diagnosis of Lewy Body Dementia (LBD) in writing. As he told me thought Parkinson's disease was the correct diagnosis on our first appointment at Swanage Hospital, he must have revised it after our second appointment at Poole Hospital. We can forget about Alzheimer's disease; we can forget about Parkinson's disease. LBD has elements of both according to my recent reading, the hallucinations, the paranoid delusions and the frequent mood changes are specifically LBD.

In retrospect, we would have liked to have been told of this diagnosis and given some advice by the Community Mental Health Team on how Jeanne's case was likely to evolve.

I can only conclude that because Jeanne was in the care home, the team decided it could be left until she was back home.

She was in safe hands for sure, but some thought for her family would have been appreciated. A book or pamphlet about LBD, advising us of some of the common difficulties and how to deal with them would have been useful. The NHS seems to have a lot of good literature for most serious and incurable conditions but I could find nothing on LBD. That is precisely why I have written this book.

During the afternoon visit to the care home, Jeanne was positively buoyant. None of us could believe how well she was talking and walking.

This is one of the remarkable things about LBD. The patient can fluctuate from one emotional extreme to another without any obvious external stimulus. I have mentioned this several times, I know. That is no reason not to mention it again.

The mood was sustained sufficiently for me to get a phone call from her at seven-thirty that evening. Nothing wrong, no complaints: just to say goodnight and that she loved me. Wonderful. I slept well that night.

Wednesday 26 August 2105

We have exchanged contracts on the sale of our house and purchase of the apartment. There is no going back for any of the parties involved.

The call came mid-afternoon and I rushed immediately to the care home to tell Jeanne. She is thrilled. So am I! Now the priority is to get the move completed as soon as possible, so that we can be together again.

Tuesday 1 September 2015

This is a bit like being in the middle lane on a motorway, with the traffic on either side of me going at varying speeds, with different intentions and differing levels of competence. The outside lane is our imminent move, the inside lane is the health of my beloved Jeanne; my middle lane is trying to keep both on course with the main objective of getting her out of the care home and back with me in the middle lane, so that, eventually, we can merge with the outside lane. We will then resume our life together and carry on in a way that passes as normal.

The moving house lane was flowing nicely; more easily than any of our previous six moves. The inside lane was very erratic. I never failed to visit her each morning and afternoon but Jeanne's thought processes were becoming less predictable by the hour. Sometimes she was buoyant, sometimes depressed. Sometimes she was pleased to see me; at other times, she looked at me with suspicion. The most taxing things to deal with were the delusions, especially the paranoid delusions. If she heard the staff laughing she was convinced they were laughing at her.

It was around this time I became aware of her difficulties with a runny nose and her reliance on an ever-present box of tissues, some of which she used to wipe her nose, but most of them she just fiddled with until they disintegrated. Sometimes she seemed to be trying to fold them in a particular pattern. It is no exaggeration to say I was having to buy a new box at least every other day, sometimes more often than that.

Wednesday 2 September 2015

Last night I sent separate, but identical, emails to Jonathan, Lizzie and Sarah. I have been concerned that in my present confused and confusing lifestyle I have been giving conflicting messages about my long-term plans for Jeanne.

Clearly, she does not enjoy life in the care home. She might well be happier in upmarket Bournemouth but this would preclude visits twice a day for sure and even once a day would be hard to maintain. The bigger issue is how long I could afford to pay their prices because I doubt if Social Services will allow her to stay there.

I am quite definite that I want her back home with me as soon as the move as taken place. When she is settled in, I shall arrange for paid outside carers to come in every day to get her up and dressed, and the reverse procedure at the end of the day.

I shall also need carers to sit in with her, from time to time, so that I can do other things without it seeming as though I am juggling to keep an unmanageable number of balls in the air. Without this help, my eventual breakdown is almost guaranteed. But I haven't mentioned any of this to Jeanne yet. She won't like it for sure.

Thursday 3 September 2015

Today we had the long-awaited visit of the consultant psychiatrist. He came to see her at the care home at 9.00am and it went better than I had hoped. He has given the care home a prescription for Rivastigmine to help her with her mental difficulties. He agrees that staying in the care home until we move will minimise her stress levels and it will also enable the staff to monitor her response to the Rivastigmine. We will receive a copy of his report in due course.

A representative of Social Services was due at the care home at 11.00am. She was 20 minutes late, of little help and left me a packet of almost unreadable leaflets.

At 3.00pm I had a call from another branch of Social Services to talk about what allowances we could claim. He was polite, on top of his job and got to the point very quickly: to paraphrase – we have too much money to claim anything!

CHAPTER TEN

Friday 4 September 2015

Today was the best day for a while. With the approval of the psychiatrist and the care home, I picked Jeanne up at 11.00am and brought her home for lunch and the rest of the day, taking her back in time for her evening meal.

She was in sparkling form and we had a lovely day together, until I had to take her back at five o'clock. But even this wasn't too difficult when she knew we would be doing the same every day from now on. It is also possible that the Rivastigmine is helping her. There's no way of knowing.

Monday 7 September 2015

Slight change of plan today. I had to clear a load of stuff out of the loft, most of which went to the dump. I picked Jeanne up after lunch, in time for Sarah to do her hair. She was a bit down: she thinks some patients at the home are talking about her and there were complaints about inadequate care. The paranoia is creeping back, just when I was thinking the Rivastigmine might getting on top of it.

Wednesday 9 September 2015

Back to 11.00am pick-up for Jeanne, yesterday and today. She was much better both days until I was taking her back for tea today when she said that I'd better not pick her up tomorrow. Why not, for heaven's sake? She said that she had heard 'the men' saying they didn't like me. They said that next time they see you – they are going to 'get' you.

Paranoia is alive and well, but I was touched that she was worried for me.

Friday 11 September 2015

I was telling Jeanne this morning that moving day is only a week away, that soon we shall be living together again in our new home. She is convinced it is all going to fall through.

Yesterday she told me the worst part of being in the care home. It was knowing that every evening I was out having dinner with another woman – whom she named. This disease is a shocker. I could say nothing to convince her of my fidelity.

Now it all becomes clear. This explains her random evening phone calls, for reasons that seemed a bit spurious and which I assumed were part of her cognitive impairment. She was checking up on me. Her paranoia had convinced her that I wasn't to be trusted, that I was having an affair. Some of the time she believed that was the sole reason that she was in the care home.

As I thought it through, I realised these ideas had been troubling her for some time. It explained why she was anxiously waiting for me by the back door when I'd popped down town, or how she couldn't understand why I didn't want to go with her and Sarah to the garden centre.

My having an affair is all that made sense to her tortured, paranoid mind. I have never given her any cause to doubt me. I have never even had the mildest of flirtations, never mind any sort of extra-marital affair. Such a temptation has never occurred to me;

no woman could possibly have taken her place in my life.

My whole life has been dedicated to her and her alone. For her to finish up like this is destroying me – just as I am getting excited about having her home again. I can no longer feel cross with her: all I have is searing sympathy for a lovely woman who did nothing to deserve this dreadful disease.

I refused to let the paranoia destroy the excitement of moving and having her back with me, where she belongs.

Wednesday 16 September 2015

Only two days to go now. At midday, I took Jeanne to Swanage Hospital. It was the final appointment with her geriatric consultant. He thought she looked well. He is handing all her future care to the psychiatrist and his Mental Health Care Team, but will always be available if needed.

Thursday 17 September 2015

All the ends are coming together. The removal firm came today to start packing as much as they could to save time tomorrow. The rest of us worked like dogs! Jeanne had to stay at the home today and she was surprisingly OK about it. I popped down to see her earlier this evening to give her a progress report – and there was no mention of 'the other woman'.

And so, to bed: the last time in this house which has been our home since 2006.

Friday 18 September 2015

MOVING DAY! It went like a charm: no legal hold ups, apart from the vendor's solicitors being at lunch when our solicitor was ready to complete. But they were soon back, and in no time, I had the keys to our new home.

> *The removal company made easy work of what was quite tricky: the flat is on the first floor with access by a two-flight staircase, or a lift designed with only people in mind. They were away soon after five so that I could report progress to Jeanne before joining everyone at Sarah's house for a family takeaway – and the odd glass of wine!*
>
> *My first night in our new home . . .*

Tomorrow my support team, otherwise known as the family, is arriving at the crack of dawn, or soon after, so we can get the place ready for me to bring Jeanne home on Sunday. I am thrilled: I just know it is going to work out.

Saturday 19 September 2015

The team beavered away all day. By mid-afternoon it seemed like a home; all it needs now to complete the picture is the arrival of my little lady. When I dropped in to see her at the end of the day she was still certain that her joining me was going to fall through. Absolutely no way!

Sunday 20 September 2015

Her misgivings are now behind her. When I arrived at the care home at 10.00am she was having a nice cup of tea with one of the senior staff who had been helping her pack ready to leave. I was so grateful because I thought the packing process would delay our leaving for at least an hour.

One small problem: the care home had forgotten to renew Jeanne's prescription and we were short of one of the key items. Luckily, they were able to lend us some, to be replaced once we had received the prescription.

But never mind all that. Jeanne seemed so relaxed, and we were in the car and away before half-past ten.

Later that day

She seems happy but, not unnaturally, a bit overwhelmed. I made us coffee so that she could take everything in slowly.

Before this dreadful disease took hold of her she would have been rushing around, diving into cupboards and planning where everything would go. But she doesn't seem troubled by her new environment. She is sitting in her own chair and seems to be taking everything in – but the box of tissues is never far away. It is almost like a comfort blanket.

As she becomes accustomed to her environment her old self returns to the scene for a while. She starts to make occasional suggestions: for instance, she would like some net curtains, and could the window blind be lower. Only little things, but encouraging nonetheless.

I had made her favourite cottage pie for lunch. She finds it one of the easier things to manage with her deteriorating motor skills.

Then I showed her our bedroom and how I had laid it out for her.

The room is L-shaped with a nice double wardrobe for her clothes, with mirror-doors, and a conveniently placed window. This leg of the 'L', I said, would be her personal space. It was set up with a pretty white

> *wickerwork table and chair for her dressing table*
> *with a five-drawer dressing chest alongside, for all*
> *her bits and bobs.*

In an earlier time, she would have loved it! Now she just accepts it.

Monday 21 September 2015

The first morning in our new home after the first night together for several weeks, I had forgotten how slow the getting up process can be. During the moving period, I had reverted to my old quick-fire way of getting things done; now I have to slow down, and be patient. We had breakfast at ten to eleven. The purchasers of our house called on us with some chocolates as a moving-in present. They are nice people but we met them in the visitors' lounge because there are unopened boxes everywhere in the apartment.

After lunch, we had to go downtown to order the missing prescription, and to buy some thank you cards for a great number of people who have done so much to help.

Tuesday 22 September 2015

Our night was slightly disturbed by a few paranoid delusions. It seems that her suspicions of the care home staff are becoming transferred to our fellow residents here. Oh, dear! But she doesn't seem seriously troubled at the moment. Time for crossed fingers; there is little else I can do.

> *This made me realise that the requests for the kitchen*
> *blind to be lower and to have net curtains at all the*
> *windows were less to do with design considerations*
> *and more to stop 'them' from spying on us.*

A day of serious unpacking followed. By the time Sarah arrived to do her Mum's hair, there were still fourteen unopened boxes in the dining room. I haven't counted the ones in the bedroom and hall yet.

Wednesday 23 September 2015

That was a much better night. Jeanne said that, when she woke in the middle of the night, she couldn't wait to see me in the morning. A far cry from my 'imposter days'. The morning routine seems slower than ever. My little lady can do little without assistance and rarely has any idea of what to do next. But, once she was settled in a comfy chair, I was able to start work on the pile of unopened boxes.

Friday 25 September 2015

Boxes, boxes, boxes! For two solid days. The problem was less about unpacking them and more about where to put all the things that came out. We have less cupboard space here, and we both have too many clothes.

Saturday 26 September 2015

It will be a long time before we are completely straight but I decided we could treat the day like a normal Saturday. Jonathan and Tracey came in for coffee and after lunch we drove out to Corfe Castle, followed by ice cream at the view point.

Sunday 27 September 2015

Last night we had umpteen 'loo calls' and, of course, I have to be alert all the time and ready to help if necessary. Then, early morning, the paranoid delusions started troubling her again. Some of them are so ridiculous it is hard not to get cross but, of course, she can't help it. I just have to be patient, but it is very hard.

Monday 28 September 2015

That was a much better night. A few bouts of paranoia soon after waking but we got to breakfast reasonably quickly. Shortly after, she fell over a rubbish bag in the dining room and banged her head on the wall. Nothing serious but she finds it hard to take things in her stride. But it was forgotten by the time Sarah came for coffee, after which we all went down to the laundry room in the basement to check out the washing machines and tumble driers, by doing a small wash. All seems pretty straightforward and I think I shall be able to cope.

Tuesday 29 September 2015

A weird start to the day. A completely imaginary 'loo accident' in the night got her off on the wrong foot. She has gone into a rather worrying version of sphinx mode, but with her eyes closed most of the time. She needs support when she walks, which she is doing with little shuffling steps, and she needs constant reassurance.

She has been withdrawn all day. I am very worried for and about her

By this time, I had been hoping to talk with one of the companies who provide daily visiting carers but Jeanne's mind was far too fragile to introduce such an idea.

Wednesday 30 September 2015

This morning I remembered the Quetiapine. I spoke to someone at the Community Mental Health Team and they have suggested we drop it until next Monday, then report back to them. I told her that I was going to make this call. When it was finished she went ballistic, and remained withdrawn and miserable all day.

I am heartbroken. I am falling apart. Finally, I have accepted that I am losing my lifetime companion. There is nothing I can do. There is no way back.

Thursday 1 October 2015

Unexpectedly, she improved before bedtime and, to my huge relief, we said goodnight on much better terms.

Then at 1.00am she was very agitated. She had been to the loo and was convinced other people were present. I gave her a Lorazepam which settled her until 5.00am when she was even worse. She was physically resistant to my attempts to help her and finally fell when I let go of her to put my glasses on.

I had reached the end of my tether: I couldn't manage alone. I had to call Sarah and Paul. They were with me in minutes. I spoke to the Mental Health Team again and they attributed Jeanne's behaviour to feelings of inadequacy. All they could suggest was a 'care in the home' package. I put the phone down, utterly despondent.

CHAPTER ELEVEN

Friday 2 October 2015

My darling Jeanne is in Poole Hospital.

With the help of Sarah, Paul and Jonathan we struggled through yesterday while her condition deteriorated to the point where we used the Careline pull cord. Careline called 999 and a paramedic was here within minutes.

He made a preliminary assessment but said he was unable to help. He said that we needed a doctor and immediately rang our GP surgery himself.

The young doctor was here sooner than we had any reason to hope. She rapidly established that Jeanne had yet another urinary tract infection. Although she could write a prescription for that, she felt the level of care Jeanne needs would be better provided in hospital. If we agreed, she could admit her with immediate effect. The only question was whether we were going to drive ourselves or would we like hospital transport? Knowing the struggle earlier in the day in just getting her to the bathroom I opted for the hospital transport. Six hours later it arrived.

There was no alternative; we realised that. Jeanne seemed to have no objections.

She was actually more relaxed than she had been for ages. I put this down to my usual explanation: she understood hospitals and knew they would make the right decisions for her. We sat together on the sofa, holding hands or with my arms around her, and talked about the past and about our family and how lucky we were to have them.

When the crew arrived, she allowed them to take her by wheelchair to the ambulance. I kissed her bye-bye and said I would be at the hospital as soon as visitors are allowed in. So here I am waiting for Sarah to pick me up after lunch. I can scarcely wait to see her sitting up in bed and taking notice.

Later that day

I am back home, and feeling utterly dejected; I had such high hopes of the effect the hospital would have on her. It was devastating to see how she had deteriorated overnight. The little old lady, who used to be Jeanne, was asleep the whole time we were there and not looking at all well. She seemed scarcely aware that we had come to see her. The Staff Nurse said that she was probably delirious from the fever caused by the infection, but went on to say that it might also be a worsening of the LBD and that a CT scan had been ordered.

Monday 5 October 2015

Absolutely no change over the weekend. I was called by a physiotherapist at the hospital this morning to who wanted to talk about Jeanne's mobility, and her general awareness. It is quite obvious from the way the physio spoke that there has been no improvement overnight.

I have a bit of a backlog of things that must be done so Sarah went in on her own today. There has been no significant change and it is beginning to look that when Jeanne leaves hospital, it will be to a care home.

When she went off last week I imagined it would be for a few days. Now? Who knows? My optimism has drained away. I am lost, out of control and hating it!

Tuesday 6 October 2015

Today I went single-handed to the hospital. Jeanne was much the same but the Staff Nurse said that she had eaten rather more today, which she regarded as a good sign. Shortly after, I saw a doctor; I think she said that she was a Registrar and not in overall charge of the case. But she was able to tell me the plan that was being drawn up for Jeanne.

They expect her treatment in Poole Hospital to be for a further two weeks. By then she should be well enough to be discharged to a care home. A social worker would be added to the care team to select a suitable care home and make all the necessary arrangements for the transfer. There will be a meeting in the next day or two. A little optimism has returned. I am looking forward to the meeting.

Thursday 8 October 2015

There was no obvious improvement in Jeanne when we visited yesterday. This morning the social worker phoned me to talk about paying for the care home.

I shall have to pay until I run out of money but she was unable to quote any figures. Somebody from a different department would do that.

The location of the care home will be arranged by the 'brokerage team' who will negotiate the best value for money – once the care package has been agreed by the clinical staff.

Saturday 10 October 2015

Meanwhile things are still going on in the background. Everybody is helping me, whenever they can, to get the flat organised. There are countless other things that need attention. Today it was the matter of the Attendance

Allowance, which I have discovered is mine by right – and I've never got around to claiming it. It has been an hour or two of filling in a form with a lot of damn-fool questions. Tonight, we are having a family meal out in an attempt to cheer ourselves up.

Sunday 11 October 2015

Lizzie was a little ahead of me in getting to the hospital today. She had downloaded Bing Crosby and Grace Kelly singing 'True Love' from the film 'High Society'. It was high in the charts when I came home from Libya in 1956 and we had adopted it as 'our tune'. Lizzie played it against Jeanne's ear which made her smile and look happy. When I arrived, she was giving her Mum her lunch, spoonful at a time, like feeding a baby. It is pitiful. I can scarcely bear to watch her deterioration.

Now I am home. Lizzie has gone back to Daventry, for work tomorrow. I am feeling forlorn and utterly helpless. There is nothing I can do! The only faint glimmer light is the meeting of the care team tomorrow, to discuss the way forward.

Monday 12 October 2015

That was a very good meeting. Jeanne's consultant was in the chair. She is convinced that Jeanne is suffering from delirium caused by the sudden change of circumstances. She anticipates that it will clear in about two weeks when she should be able to go into a care home. Carers coming into our home on a daily basis would not provide the necessary level of care she will need.

At this point, I asked the consultant the question that needs answering.

"Are we looking at end-of-life care?"

Her reply was somehow reassuring but confirmed what I suspected. It probably is end-of-life but there is no knowing how long it will be. Her guess is that it will be months rather than weeks.

The social worker explained that a 'brokerage team' would start working on finding a care home providing the appropriate level of care at a price acceptable to Social Services. She verified that, if I choose to buy Jeanne a higher level of care, when I run out of money they will move her to a home acceptable to them. In my opinion, this is not in Jeanne's best interests so we must start at the level of care they are prepared to fund. I was assured that the care would be totally adequate. Where it will be, is a significant question. We won't know this until the brokerage team has done its work. My concern, of course, is maintaining sufficient access that all of us can visit with reasonable frequency – in all weathers.

Thursday 15 October 2015

I have been busy keeping on top of everything with the help of the rest of the team.

I have spoken to the CMHT to confirm that, while Jeanne is in hospital, they play only a watching role in her care.

I've had a dental job done myself, and had my annual diabetic eyes screening. These things go on even though we are far more occupied with the bigger issue.

Today I came away from the hospital with some foreboding. There was a sign over Jeanne's bed: NIL BY MOUTH. I am not really surprised. She has been more or less comatose for the past few days.

Friday 16 October 2015

This morning was emotional. I have been clearing up things in our bedroom which were as Jeanne left them on the night she went into hospital – as though she will be coming back. She won't. The best I can hope for is a care home – and she hated that.

Back to reality. Down to the laundry room: washing on, then back down to transfer it to a tumble dryer. Then the ironing.

Soon after, Sarah and Paul stopped by on the way back from the hospital. A doctor has been trying to call me: if things become critical in the middle of the night, would I want to be woken up. The answer they gave on my behalf was a definite yes. They were, of course, right. But this is absolutely bloody dreadful!

Tuesday 20 October 2015

When she went into the care home on the 8 August, I recorded it as being the worst day of my life. It seems like a picnic now.

The days go by and, despite everything, I am managing to appear fairly normal. Today Jonathan and Tracey visited the hospital while I went out to do a bit of drawing to get away from the anticipation of the inevitable. Tracey leaned over Jeanne and told her everyone sent their love. She opened her eyes and smiled briefly.

Wednesday 21 October 2015

I felt a bit sub-standard on waking up: I am not sleeping well enough. There was no change at the hospital. The Staff Nurse said that Jeanne's 'care pathway' is definitely 'end-of-life'. She said that my darling had become very frail in the last day or two. They are doing everything to keep her comfortable. We can visit at any time of the night or day – and we can park for free if we take our ticket to the car park office.

Thursday 22 October 2015

I sat down to do the accounts and the phone rang.

I knew before picking it up that it was the call I had been dreading.

The Staff Nurse said that Jeanne slipped away about three o'clock this afternoon.

I am completely and utterly distraught.

It is impossible to prepare oneself for the actuality of this moment.

She was my life, my love, my everything. Even in the darkest moments of these last few weeks I adored her.

Later that day

I managed to hold it all together while I called Jonathan, Lizzie and Sarah.

Sarah took me on a brief visit to the hospital where we did all we had to and where we met up with Jonathan and Tracey. Sarah brought me back to my flat.

A few hours ago, this was our flat; now it is mine.

Now, I am on my own and feel completely numb.

I knew it was going to happen.

For her sake, I wanted it to happen. She had suffered enough.

But that doesn't make it any easier.

CHAPTER TWELVE

November 2015: one month later

Sadly, with Lewy Body Disease there can be no happy ending. The best I could hope for was what we achieved: a memorable and fitting closure to the life of the beautiful person who meant so much to me and to so many other people.

The numbness following the final phone call from Poole Hospital insulated me from the worst of my emotions as we dealt with all the practical things that followed the death of my darling Jeanne.

The essential component of my support system is the all day, every day, unconditional love of my family. I have always valued our 'corporate strength'. Any one of us, or all of us, can be relied on, in any sort of crisis to deliver what is necessary. We are also good at being outwardly cheery, even under the worst imaginable circumstances. Behind the scenes we all had our private and less private meltdowns, but I think we can be proud of being a family that can cope.

During the first day or two, Lizzie was with me as we set about sorting Jeanne's clothes and effects into three piles: a) pass on to the family, b) give to Sue Ryder, c) dump! It definitely needed a woman's touch, but it was heavy with emotional overtones for us both.

The formal necessities needed a more corporate approach. Once we received the death certificate from the Hospital, we saw the Poole Registrar, the Undertakers, the Rector to plan the funeral service, the Grand Hotel to arrange for a buffet afterwards, the florists and the local paper for an obituary notice. All were brilliant: we didn't have to worry about a thing.

Family and friends filled St Mary's Church in Swanage with love. The funeral service was both stylish and beautiful: a fitting tribute our lovely Jeanne, Mum and Nana. She would have given it full marks. Jonathan did the Bible reading, Rick gave his personal eulogy, the music was well-chosen and the Rector added his own special touch to make it truly memorable. The committal at the Godlingston Cemetery in Swanage was for the family only.

The Grand Hotel lived up to expectations. In spite of our personal grief, we were able to circulate amongst our family and friends, some of whom had travelled appreciable distances to be with us and to pay their respects to this gracious person who meant so much to us all.

January 2016: three months later

I have survived Christmas and the first three months without her. Life will never be the same but there is no value in wallowing in grief and feeling sorry for myself.

Organising the apartment to meet my needs has kept me occupied. It took very few weeks of winter weather to find that the storage heaters installed by McArthy & Stone were well past their useful life. I have bought new electric radiators of the latest design that are working efficiently. Only time will tell how cost-effective they will be. Gas central heating was out of the question: there is no gas in the building

Luke now has his picture of the fishermen's beach in Swanage. I managed to get it finished in time for Christmas. He likes it – thank goodness! I have several other pictures planned but painting is a solitary occupation. I need to get out more!

April 2016: six months later

Early in the new year I had one of my better ideas. It was acknowledged by everyone, especially me, that I was useless at finding my way round Poole Hospital. The others were better than me, but none of us found it easy – it is a rabbit warren of a building. The staff are friendly and will always try to help patients and visitors, when asked, by giving directions but they rarely have the time to do any more – and they don't necessarily know some of the more obscure destinations themselves. Why not couple this problem with my need to get out more? Why not volunteer to be a hospital guide?

I found an application form on the hospital website, filled it in and popped it in the post, expecting an enthusiastic 'When can you start?' letter by return. Far from it! The reply was 'Sorry, we don't take volunteers from outside the Poole area.'

Taking no for an answer is not one of my stronger characteristics. Persuading people to my point of view probably is. I spoke with the Volunteers' Lead that same day. Apparently volunteers from further afield usually forget to factor in the travelling time and many give up after a few weeks. I'm not sure exactly what I said to cause the lady's resistance to crumble so effectively; probably it was sheer volume of words. I can go on a bit when necessary.

Going through all the hoops to satisfy the NHS that I am a suitable candidate has taken until now. I have just attended the April Induction Meeting for new employees which, surprisingly, covered all levels of staff from volunteers, clerical staff, nurses, and junior doctors to consultants. The more senior the inductee, the longer they had to stay. From my lowly position, I escaped soon after lunchtime; the consultants were scheduled to be there until lunch time the following day.

I am waiting to hear when I am to start.

October 2016: one year later

While I was waiting for the call to start working I spent several mornings just wandering around the hospital, working out the general layout of the buildings. By the time I started, I had the basic framework in my mind.

The first working day was 26 April when I reported to the Outpatients Department. My job was to meet and greet patients, make sure they were in the right clinic and help them use the self-check-in when necessary. There were other duties that didn't amount to much. The clinical and clerical staff were all very nice but, to be honest, I found it all rather boring and time dragged. In consequence, I gradually expanded my job well beyond Outpatients to include the corridors to and from the department where I found patients and visitors looking as though they might need help. Giving them a friendly greeting, asking if they need help and, when necessary (which is almost always) getting them to the right place is exactly right for me, and hugely appreciated by the patients.

I am very happy now, working on Monday and Thursday afternoons each week. There are several others doing similar work and we have banded together informally as a team. The time flies and the amount of walking necessary is keeping me very fit. I have an app on my mobile phone that measures the distances I walk doing this job. It is consistently in the region of three to four miles per shift.

In the summer, I was visited by a friend of mine from Ireland. I have known him since the early 1970s and we have many interests in common. His first name is also Brian so, to avoid any confusion, I will call him by his surname, as I often do in real life. I was telling McIvor how I had tried to find a book on Lewy Body Dementia, from a carer's point of view, without success, and how much one was needed to give advice on the sort of things that might be expected.

"You should do it yourself," was his immediate reaction, "you have the necessary skills, and have been through it all." A hundred reasons why not buzzed through my head, when I heard myself saying:

"Are you throwing down the gauntlet?"

"I am throwing down the gauntlet!" This sounds better in his Irish accent.

"Right! You'll have the first draft by the end of August."

Did I really say that?

It is a great deal harder than I expected; and I expected it to be almost impossible. I've revised the deadline from the end of August to Christmas, but I am working on it. I mustn't take the soft option, and duck out. It will be written.

October 2017: two years later

I finally got the first draft to Jonathan, Lizzie and Sarah for their comments on 8 May this year. I also sent a copy to Luke for his professional advice on facts and another to Rick, a CBT specialist, for his input. One further copy to McIvor, as you would expect. He started the whole thing.

Comments, corrections of fact and spelling mistakes all found their way back. I did a second edit, and a third, added this final chapter, compiled the additional notes and spent a few days on spit and polish before sending it to the publishers. They have done their work.

So, dear reader, as we say in Dorset: "YER TIZ!" I hope you find it helpful.

EPILOGUE

Although a member of the Church of England by upbringing, I am not a deeply spiritual person. I am best defined as a Christian agnostic who believes there are things beyond the reach of human senses, that we are not meant to understand.

I thought Jeanne would want to leave this earthly life wearing her engagement ring, which we chose together, and a cameo brooch I sent her for her twenty-first birthday when I was serving in Libya, both of which she treasured. Her actual wedding ring had long since worn away and had been replaced by one belonging to her mother. She had stopped wearing her engagement ring for fear of it going the same way.

Lizzie and I searched everywhere for them. We emptied her two jewellery boxes and spread the contents out on the bed. Neither was there. Deeply disappointed, I reasoned that she had probably thrown them away in anger in the last weeks of her illness, when her paranoid delusions led her to believe that I was having an affair. Lizzie had to go back to Daventry the next day.

Two days later I decided to have just one more look. I opened the first box. The engagement ring was sitting right on top! I was thrilled. I sent a delighted text to Lizzie straight away. I could hardly dare to open the other box. It was there! The cameo brooch was sitting right on top again. I was happy. I had closure.

Months later, I lost the ring Jeanne gave me on our Golden Wedding Anniversary. It had been on my finger when I went to the Swanage shops; when I got home it was gone. I searched everywhere and rang each of the shops I'd visited, Nothing.

The next day I was off to work at the hospital. I have a photo of Jeanne just inside the front door. I stopped by and spoke to her, as I often do.

"Come on, you're good at finding rings – please find my wedding ring!"

When I got home the ring was lying on the carpet, just inside the door, where I couldn't possibly miss it.

I have drawn my own conclusions from this. I invite you to draw yours . . .

FURTHER INFORMATION

Lewy Body Dementia is also known as Dementia with Lewy Bodies, and Lewy Body Disease or by their acronyms of DLB and LBD. They are all the same illness.

All the signs and symptoms that characterised my wife's illness are mentioned in the text but there is are several websites where additional information can be found. All of them stress that no two cases of LBD are identical.

This list is by no means complete but covers the main points.

Alzheimers Society (www.alzheimers.org.uk)

The Lewy Body Society (www.lewybody.org)

National Health Service
(www.nhs.uk.org/dementia-with-lewy-bodies)

OTHER USEFUL SITES

Lasting Power of Attorney

(**www.gov.uk>power-of-attorney**)

This is the only site you need, and it is very complete. It tells you all you need to know and provides the forms for you download and details of how to submit them to the Office of the Public Guardian who have to register your LPA. There is a cost for OPG registration. The current cost can be found on the website.

Attendance Allowance

(**www.gov.uk>attendance-allowance**)

This site tells you everything you need to know.